Hospital automation And Information Management

Hospital Automation And Information Management

C. Charles

ANMOL PUBLICATIONS PVT. LTD.
NEW DELHI - 110 002 (INDIA)

ANMOL PUBLICATIONS PVT. LTD.

H.O.: 4374/4B, Ansari Road, Darya Ganj
New Delhi-110 002 (India)
Ph.: 23278000, 23261597

B.O.: 1015, Ist Main Road, BSK IIIrd Stage
IIIrd Phase, IIIrd Block
Bangalore - 560 085 (Karnataka)
Ph: 080-41723429, Tel/Fax: 080-2672 3604
Visit us at: www.anmolpublications.com

Hospital Automation and Information Management

First Published, 2008

ISBN 978-81-261-3287-4

PRINTED IN INDIA

Printed at Mehra Offset Press, Delhi.

Contents

Preface

Today, there is a strong desire for customer satisfaction in health services. Benchmarking needs to be implemented for hospital managers to be better prepared in identifying gaps in management, to be in a better positioned to determine training needs and to be able to identify those areas in which to apply more cost effective practices in performance. These will, in turn, aid in improving the quality of management and services. If the hospitals, the government and the information technology vendors come together with an agreed framework regarding the use of the technology to improve the quality of the patient care, then one can see smiles on the ailing faces, calmness in the working nurses, freshness in the technology savvy doctors, and cash flow fulfillment in the anxious management. According to a study conducted by American Medical Association, 94 per cent of the US physicians use computers in their practice, and 79 per cent use the Internet or an online network compared to 80 per cent and 61 per cent averages for the 15 countries in the European Union. Cent percent of doctors in Finland and the Netherlands are reported to use computers and an online network. According to a survey from Harris Interactive Inc., 26 per cent of America's practicing physicians used hand-held devices for professional and personal activities in 2001, up from 15 per cent in 1999. Harris Interactive estimates that 50 per cent of the country's physicians will be using the devices by 2005. But that could change markedly if insurers, employers, hospitals and other providers mandate physician usage

Information consists of two parts, facts and communication. It is not enough for one person to know a fact; the fact must be communicated for it to be of any value to anyone else. Forms were invented to do just that—communicate facts in a systematic manner from one party to the next. Automating forms with computers on a local area network or a wide area network allows for hospital personnel to input a patient's information once and electronically share the information from one department to another, simultaneously. Switching from a paper-based forms system to a fully automated workflow forms system or combining the two can save healthcare institution money, errors, time and even lives. The levels of an automated forms system include: electronic forms design, demand printing, typewriter replacement, intelligent forms, intelligent mail and true workflow automation. Use of pre-printed forms to manage hospital daily business processes is costly and inefficient. Manual data entry can lead to errors of interpretation. The dynamic nature of the healthcare industry demands a solution that allows changes to be implemented quickly and easily. By using OKI color and mono printers and partner software, hospitals can automate the creation, distribution and printing of forms and patient packets. Admission packets can be assembled automatically, pre-populated with patient's demographics information and routed simultaneously to a variety of output devices such as printers, archiving systems, e-mail box and fax machines located in different departments. OKI Forms Automation is an ideal solution to enhance patient safety, improve quality of patient care and simplify regulatory compliance. A hospital's medical records department traditionally has invoked images of color-coded manila folders and unmanageable stacks of paper. With the inception of diagnosis related groups (DRGs) and the ever-increasing number of agencies seeking documentation from hospitals, the mass of paperwork has increased substantially, making it difficult for medical records to manually keep up with demands on its limited resources. Many medical records departments do not have the tools to meet the requests of hospital administrators, physicians, peer review organizations (PROs), the Joint Commission on Accreditation of Healthcare Organizations (JCAHO), third-party payers, attorneys, patients, and private utilization reviewers. These requests can severely hamper a hospital's cash flow if the institution cannot produce the documentation needed in a timely manner. Consequently, a medical records department has become a prominent component of a financially stable healthcare facility. Hospitals are realizing the importance of implementing computerized medical records systems to match computer-strong admissions departments and business offices. Health Information implies information in any form (oral, written or otherwise) that relates to the past, present or future physical or mental health of an individual. That information could be created or received by a health care provider, a health plan, a public health authority, an employer, a life insurer, a school, a university or a health care clearinghouse. All health information is protected by state and federal confidentiality laws and by privacy rules.

Any organization when automated, transforms its business processes into a near paperless system, controlling costs, saving time and thereby aiding in quick decision making and increasing the efficiency of the total system or organization. This is possible as all the information is available online at any point of time. For example, if a bank were automated, then one would know the details of the transactions of an account-holder instantly based on the unique account number of the account holder. Now the question is, when a hospital is automated will the doctor know his in-patient's condition or progress online, based on his unique identifying number or code and give instructions online? Is the information pertaining to the patient's previous visits, surgeries, diseases, allergies, lab reports, medication, etc., available at his fingertips for analyzing and providing proper medication? Though most would say 'yes', the fact is, it is not happening in the hospitals in India with an exception of a handful of corporate health care providers who claim that they have almost transformed their hospitals into paperless and filmless systems. Many hospitals are being automated, but the scope of their usage is limited to administrative functions. Most of the hospitals, which claim that they have computerized their business processes, have only billing, finance and accounts and to a certain extent inventory either fully or partially automated. This means that only administrative staff would be using computers, leaving little or no scope for doctors in using computers for providing quality patient care.

The process of implementing a health care automation and information system begins with modeling the organization in software. The degree to which adaptation of the system to the organization is successful places an upper limit on the degree to which adoption will be successful. A mature and well-designed system will allow an organization to dictate how the software works rather than the other way around, and the system will allow for a great deal of variation in how different parts of the organization operate. Although that is the case, choices must be made about how detailed a model is necessary for a complex organization. In a very large organization, a precise model is far too expensive to be a realistic proposition. We can liken the software-modeling phase of the implementation to making a map of a geographic region. The more details there are, the more topography represented, the larger the map must be, and the longer it will take to create it. Its size may make it impractical to wield as a tool; its expense in time and resources may make it impossible to afford. A pocket-sized map giving a general but accurate knowledge of the terrain is much more useful and can be created in a reasonable amount of time, making it also affordable. It won't indicate every tree root to step over or every stream to cross, but if you know how to step over roots and cross-streams, you don't usually need that information anyway. With a health care software system, you don't need a specialized workflow or data collection form for every possible clinical presentation or registration situation. You need a few tools that encapsulate the variation in a majority of your work practices, some special tools for infrequent but important situations, and the ability to branch away from standard templates in the remaining situations. That means that you can model the large-scale features of the organization, mapping them to system functionality and tools, teach users how to handle unknown terrain, and get them using the system in a reasonable amount of time.

This publication entitled "Hospital Automation and Information Management" can be used as a reference book for current opinion and the latest developments in the field of hospital aautomation and information management.

—Editor

1

Introduction to Hospital Information Management and Automation

HEALTH MANAGEMENT INFORMATION SYSTEMS

A Quick Guide Through the Key Issues

Health management information incorporates all the data needed by policy makers, clinicians and health service users to improve and protect population health. Few countries in the world today have effective and comprehensive systems in place to gather this data.

Yet there has never been a greater need for robust health information. As the world community has turned its attention to meeting Millennium Development Goal targets, and ever increasing resources are going towards preventing and treating high burden diseases such as HIV and AIDS, tuberculosis and malaria, decision-makers need to be able to measure whether policies and programmes are working, and whether progress is being made towards the goals that have been set. Donors are also placing more emphasis on performance, linking the release of funds to performance based measures. See Structuring information and incentives to improve health.

The World Health Organisation (WHO) argues that investment in health management information systems

(HMIS) now could reap multiple benefits, including:

- — helping decision makers to detect and control emerging and endemic health problems, monitor progress towards health goals, and promote equity;
- — empowering individuals and communities with timely and understandable health-related information, and drive improvements in quality of services;
- — strengthening the evidence base for effective health policies, permitting evaluation of scale-up efforts, and enabling innovation through research;
- — improving governance, mobilising new resources, and ensuring accountability in the way they are used

Hospital Information System

A hospital information system (HIS), variously also called clinical information system (CIS) is a comprehensive, integrated information system designed to manage the administrative, financial and clinical aspects of a hospital. This encompasses paper-based information processing as well as data processing machines.

As an area of medical informatics the aim of an HIS is to achieve the best possible support of patient care and administration by electronic data processing.

It can be composed of one or few software components with specialty specific extensions as well as of a large variety of sub-systems in medical specialties (e.g. Laboratory Information System, Radiology Information System).

CISs are sometimes separated from HISs in that the former concentrate on patient- and clinical state- related data (electronic patient record) whereas the latter keeps track of administrative issues. The distinction is not always clear and there is contradictory evidence against a consistent use of both terms.

ELECTRONIC MEDICAL RECORD

Definition

An EMR facilitates:

- access of patient data by clinical staff at any given location
- accurate and complete claims processing by insurance companies
- building automated checks for drug and allergy interactions
- clinical notes
- prescriptions
- scheduling
- sending to and viewing by labs

The term has become expanded to include systems which keep track of other relevant medical information. The practice management system is the medical office functions which support and surround the electronic medical record. Although an EMR system has the potential to permit invasion of medical privacy, if security policies are monitored effectively EMRs are as secure as banking records, for example.

Electronic records in health fall under the purview of health informatics, a combination of computation and computer science and medical record keeping.

According to the Medical Records Institute, five levels of an Electronic HealthCare Record (EHCR) can be distinguished:

— The is a paper-based record with some computer-generated documents.
— The makes the documents of level 1 electronically available.
— The (EMR) restructures and optimizes the documents of the previous levels ensuring inter-operability of all documentation systems.
— The is a patient-centered record with information from multiple institutions.
— The adds general health-related information to the EPR that is not necessarily related to a disease.

Interoperability

In the United States, the development of standards for EMR interoperability is at the forefront of the national health care agenda. Without interoperable EMRs, practicing physicians, pharmacies and hospitals cannot share patient information, which is necessary for timely, patient-centered and portable care. There are currently multiple competing vendors of EHR systems, each selling a software suite that in many cases is not compatible with those of their competitors. Only counting the outpatient vendors, there are more than 25 major brands currently on the market. In 2004, President Bush created the Office of the National Coordinator for Health Information Technology (ONC), originally headed by David Brailer, in order to address interoperability issues and to establish a National Health Information Network (NHIN).

Under the ONC, Regional Health Information Organisations (RHIOs) have been estabilshed in many states in order to promote the sharing of health information. Congress is currently working on legislation to increase funding to these and similar programmes.

EMR Issues

As of 2006, adoption of EMRs and other health information technology, such as computer physician order entry (CPOE), has been minimal in the United States. Less than 10% of American hospitals have implemented health information technology, while a mere 16% of primary care physicians use EHRs. The vast majority of healthcare transactions in the United States still take place on paper, a system that has remained unchanged since the 1950s. The healthcare industry spends only 2% of gross revenues on HIT, which is meager compared to other information intensive industries such as finance, which spend upwards of 10%. The following issues are behind the slow rate of adoption:

Adding Older Records to EMRs

To attain the wide accessibility, efficiency, patient safety and cost savings promised by EMR, older paper medical records ideally should be incorporated into the patient's record. The digital scanning process involved in conversion of these physical records to EMR is an expensive, time-consuming process, which must be done to exacting standards to ensure exact capture of the content. Because many of these records involve extensive handwritten content, some of which may have been generated by different healthcare professionals over the life span of the patient, some of the content is illegible following conversion. The material may exist in any number of formats, sizes, media types and qualities, which further complicates accurate conversion. In addition, the destruction of original healthcare records must be done in a way that ensures that they are completely and confidentially destroyed. Results of scanned records are not always useable; medical surveys found that 22-25% of physicians much less satisfied with the use of scanned document images than that of regular electronic data.

Social and Organisational Barriers

According to the Agency for Healthcare Research and Quality's National Resource Center for Health Information Technology, EMR implementations follow the 80/20 rule; that is, 80% of the work of implementation must be spent on issues of change management, while only 20% is spent on technical issues related to the technology itself. Such organisational and social issues include restructuring workflows, dealing with physicians' resistance to change (or, alternatively, software engineers' evolving research in deep modeling of the physician's knowledge and workflow domains), and creating a collaborative environment that fosters communication between physicians and information technology project managers. Exemplifying this need are several highly publicized HIT implementation fiascos, including one at Cedars Sinai Medical Center in Los Angeles, in which physicians revolted and forced the administration to scrap a $34 million CPOE system.

Privacy

A major concern is adequate confidentiality of the individual records being managed electronically. According to the , roughly 150 people (from doctors and nurses to technicians and billing clerks) have access to at least part of a patient's records during a hospitalisation, and 600,000 payers, providers and other entities that handle providers' billing data have some access also. Multiple access points over an open network like the internet increases possible patient data interception. In the United States, this class of information is referred to as Personal Healthcare Information (PHI) and its management is addressed under the Health Insurance Portability and Accountability Act (HIPAA) as well as many local laws. In the European Union (EU), several Directives of the European Parliament and of the Council protect the processing and free movement of personal data, including for purposes of health care. The organisations and individuals charged with the management of this information are required to ensure adequate protection is provided and that access to the information is only by authorized parties. The growth of EHR creates new issues, since electronic data may be physically much more difficult to secure, as lapses in data security are increasingly being reported. Information security practices have been established for computer networks, but technologies like wireless computer networks offer new challenges as well.

Legal Status of EMR

Medical records, such as physician orders, exam and test reports are legal documents, which must be kept in unaltered form and authenticated by the creator.

— Digital signatures Most national and international standards accept electronic signatures. According to the American Bar Association, "A signature authenticates a writing by identifying the signer with the signed document. When the signer makes a mark in a distinctive manner, the writing becomes attributable to the signer." With proper security software, electronic authentication is more difficult to falsify than the handwritten doctor's signature. However, as the recent rise in identity theft demonstrates, no security method can totally prevent fraud, so auditing information security will contiue to be prudent when using EMR.

— Digital records such as EHR create difficulties ensuring that the content, context and structure are preserved when the records do not have a physical existence. As of 2006, national and state archives authorities are still developing open, non-proprietary technical standards for electronic records management (ERM).

Preserving Electronic Records

Under data protection legislation and the law generally responsibilty for patient records (irrespective of the form they are kept in) is always on the creator and custodian of the record, usually a health care practice or facility. The physical medical records are the property of the medical provider (or facility) that prepares them. This includes films and tracings from diagnostic imaging procedures such as x-ray, CT, PET, MRI, ultrasound, etc. The patient, however, according to HIPAA, owns the information contained within the record and has a right to view the originals, and to obtain copies under law. Additionally, those responsible for the management of the EMR are responsible to see the hardware, software and media used to manage the information remain usable and not degraded. This requires backup of the data and protection being provided to copies. It will also require the planned periodic migration of information to address concerns of media degradation from use.

Standards

Though there are few standards for modern day EMR systems as a whole, there are many standards relating to specific aspects of EHRs and EMRs. These include:

- ASTM International Continuity of Care Record - a patient health summary standard based upon XML, the CCR can be created, read and interpreted by various EHR or EMR systems, allowing easy interoperability between otherwise disparate enities.
- ANSI X12 (EDI) - A set of transaction protocols used for transmitting virtually any aspect of patient data. Has become popular in the United States for transmitting billing information, because several of the transactions became required by the Health

Insurance Portability and Accountability Act (HIPAA) for transmitting data to Medicare.

— CEN - EN13606, the European standard for the communication of information from EHR systems, and HISA, a services standard for inter-system communication in a clinical information environment.

— DICOM - a heavily used standard for representing and communicating radiology images and reporting

— HL7 - HL7 messages are used for interchange between hospital and physician record systems and between EMR systems and practice management systems; HL7 Clinical Document Architecture (CDA) documents are used to communicate documents such as physician notes and other material.

— ISO - ISO TC215 has defined the EHR, and also produced a technical specification ISO 18308 describing the requirements for EHR Architectures.

— openEHR - next generation public specifications and implementations for EHR systems and communication, based on a complete separation of software and clinical models.

Customisation

Pricing for EMR systems is highly dependent on each practice's unique needs. Because every medical practice has distinct requirements, systems usually need to be custom tailored. This is due to the majority of EMR systems being based on templates that are initially general in scope. In many cases, these templates can then be customized in co-operation with the vendor/developer to better fit a medical specialty, environment or other specified needs. There are also EMR systems available that do not use templates and therefore can be easily personalized by each individual user, for example those based on Concept Processing technology.

Caveats and Concerns

There are issues surrounding the generation and management of electronic medical records (EMRs), sometimes known as electronic health records (EHRs).

There are a two primary categories of the EMR; the "born digital" record and the scanned/imaged record.

The "born digital" record, which is information captured in a native electronic format originally is information that may be entered into a database, transcribed from an electronic tablet or notebook PC, or in some other manner captured from its inception electronically. The information is then transferred to a server or other host environment, where it is stored electronically.

The second category are records originally produced in a paper or other hardcopy form (x-ray film, photographs, etc.) that have been scanned or imaged and converted to a digital form. These records are best described as "digital format records", as their content is not able to be modified or altered (with the exception of the use of a third party software to make "overlay notations") as electronic records are. Most medical records generated preceding the year 2000 are of this category.

The process involved in conversion of these physical records to EMR is an expensive, time-consuming process, which must be done to exacting standards to ensure exact and accurate capture of the content. Because many of these records involve extensive handwritten content, some of which may have been generated by any number of healthcare professionals over the life span of the patient, there exists a high probability of some of the content being illegible following conversion. In addition, the material may exist in any number of formats, sizes, media types and qualities, which further complicates accurate conversion. Consideration should be given to developing a procedure to sample and verify images at a high ratio to determine the accuracy and usability of the scanned images prior to disposal of the physical records, if they are disposed of at all.

Further, all electronic repositories of information are subject to the need for periodic conversion and migration to ensure the formats they were captured in remain accessible over the life of the patient, and in some cases beyond, to the expected life of their heirs. Additionally, those responsible for the management of the EMR are responsible to see the hardware, software (applications) and media used to manage the information remain viable and are not subject to obsolecense or degradation. This will require generation of backup copies of the data and protection being provided to these copies in the event of damage to the primary repository. It will also require the planned periodic migration of information to address concerns of media degradation from use. These are all costly, time consuming processes that must be planned and budgeted for when making decisions to convert physical medical records to digital formats.

Another major concern is adequate protection of privacy of the individuals whose records are being managed electronically. This class of information (in the US) is referred to as Personal Healthcare Information (PHI) and its management is addressed under the Healthcare Insurance Portability and Accountability Act (HIPAA) as well as many State-specific privacy laws. The organisation/individuals charged with the management of this information are required to ensure adequate protection is provided and that access to the information is only by authorized parties.

Public Implementations

As of 2005, one of the largest projects for a national EMR is by the National Health Service (NHS) in the United Kingdom. The goal of the NHS is to have 60,000,000 patients with a centralized electronic medical record by 2010.

The Canadian province of Alberta's Alberta Netcare project is a large-scale operational EMR system.

Adoption of electronic medical records by US doctors is increasing slowly. The latest data from the National Ambulatory Medical Care Survey (NAMCS) indicate that one-quarter of office-based physicians report using fully or partially electronic medical record systems (EMR) in 2005, a 31% increase from the 18.2 percent reported in the 2001 survey. However, the survey also states that just 9.3% of these physicians actually have a "complete EMR system", with all four basic functions deemed minimally necessary for a full EMR: computerized orders for prescriptions, computerized orders for tests, reporting of test results, and physician notes. Barriers to adopting an EMR system include training, costs and complexity, as well as the lack of a national standard for interoperability among competing software options. Advocates of electronic health records hope that product certification will provide US physicians and hospitals with the assurance they need to justify significant investments in new systems. The Certification Commission for Healthcare Information Technology (CCHIT), a private nonprofit group, was funded in 2005 by the U.S. Department of Health and Human Services to develop a set of standards and certify vendors who meet them. On July 18 2006, CCHIT released its first list of 20 certified ambulatory EMR and EHR products. and then on July 31 2006, additionally announced that two further EMR and EHR products had achieved certification.

In the United States, the Department of Veterans Affairs (VA) has the largest enterprise-wide health information system that includes an electronic medical record, known as the Veterans Health Information Systems and Technology Architecture or VistA. A graphical user interface known as the Computerized Patient Record System (CPRS) allows health care providers to review and update a patient's electronic medical record at any of the VA's over 1,000 healthcare facilities. CPRS includes the ability to place orders, including medications, special procedures, x-rays, patient care nursing orders, diets, and laboratory tests.

OFFICE AUTOMATION (OA)

Policy

a. OA will be managed and acquired as Federal Information Processing (FIP) resources in accordance with:

  (1) The Paperwork Reduction Act of 1980, as amended (44 United States Code (U.S.C.) 35), and

  (2) Federal policy and regulations such as: (i) Federal Information Resources Management Regulations (FIRMR), (ii) Federal Acquisitions Regulations (FAR), (iii) Federal Information Processing Standards (FIPS) of the National Institute for Standards and Technology (NIST), and (iv) Office of Management and Budget (OMB) Circular A-130, Management of Federal Information Resources.

b. All health care facility OA systems must be compatible with existing Veteran Health Administration (VHA) information systems. They must be capable of exchanging data/text with existing VHA information systems.

(1) The Decentralized Hospital Computer Programme (DHCP) MailMan system is the preferred electronic mail system. MailMan software must be installed and utilized as the facility's primary electronic mail system.

(2) Other X.400 compliant electronic mail systems may be used on a limited basis provided that the systems are interfaced and that proper procurement exemptions are obtained.

c. VHA will plan comprehensively for all OA system activities. Acquisition planning for all OA and other Automated Data Processing (ADP) will be integrated to maximise the use of existing and future technical resources.

d. OA procurements must follow the same procedures as other ADP equipment and, therefore, must be justified by a requirements analysis so that management approval or disapproval can be based upon objective evaluations. The requirements analysis, as described in MP-6, Part I, Chapter 7, Appendix A, will include a detailed cost/benefit analysis commensurate with the size and scope of the procurement. In addition.

e. Acquisition of OA resources will be included and justified through the VHA automated facility ADP planning package (PlanMan).

f. In order to meet agency strategic planning interoperability goals, all OA equipment must be upgradable to comply with the Open Systems Interconnection (OSI) communications protocol suite as they become industry standards as required.

g. Dissimilar OA systems used within a facility must be able to transfer files electronically without the need to physically transport any media.

h. All stand-alone OA work stations must be capable of being configured to access and fully operate with existing VHA information systems.

l Shared logic and shared storage OA systems and printers must be capable of being accessible from any existing VHA information system.

j. To promote VA's goal of interconnectivity/ interoperability, any terminal used must be able to access any other major VA system.

k. There will be no vendor-specific requirements included in OA justifications.

l. Any requests for exceptions to policy must be specifically justified in PlanMan and all applicable acquisition requests.

Purpose

The purpose of this chapter is to establish policy and guidance governing the procurement of OA equipment and software which will function as a vital component of the Department of Veterans Affairs (VA) health care information systems.

Definitions

a. Interconnectivity. Interconnectivity is the ability of dissimilar computer systems to physically connect to each other.

b. Interoperability. Interoperability involves the ability of dissimilar computer systems to fully interact with each other. Interoperability implies a higher level of integration than interconnectivity.

c. OA. OA includes, but is not limited to:

(1) Word processing,

(2) Spreadsheets,

(3) Graphics,

(4) Electronic mail,

(5) Appointment calendars, and

(6) Telephone directories.

d. OSI. OSI is a collection of international standards developed by the International Standards Organisation for the promotion of interconnectivity and interoperability of multi-vendor computer environments.

e. PlanMan.

The PlanMan software package provides the process by which health care facilities can enter data for their 5-year ADP plans.

Responsibilities

a. OA planning will be conducted consistent with VHA policy for ADP planning. All VHA OA initiatives will be in the facility's ADP Plan.

b. The Director, Medical Information Resource Management Office (MIRMO), is responsible for the review of all OA-related plans and/or requests for VHA and for approval/disapproval of individual facility's OA requests.

c. The Information Systems Center (ISC) Directors are responsible for reviewing the facility OA plans and equipment requests and submitting comments and recommendations to the Director, MIRMO.

d. Each VHA field facility is responsible for:

(1) Preparing and submitting OA-related plans or requests to their respective ISC for review;

(2) Updating the facility's ADP Plan annually with appropriate OA initiatives; and

(3) Submission of OA acquisition requests for OA initiatives shall follow the same procedures for other ADP equipment as defined in: (i) Chapter 2, (ii) MP-6, Part I, Chapter 3, "VA Information Systems Planning," and (iii) MP-6, Part I, Chapter 7, "Acquisition of Information Resources."

AUTOMATED MEDICATION DISPENSING DEVICES

In the 1980s, automated dispensing devices appeared on the scene, a generation after the advent of unit-dose dispensing. The invention and production of these devices brought hopes of reduced rates of medication errors, increased efficiency for pharmacy and nursing staff, ready availability of medications where they are most often used (the nursing unit or inpatient ward), and improved pharmacy inventory and billing functions. Although the capacity of such systems to contribute to patient safety appears great, surprisingly few studies have evaluated the clinical impact of these devices.

Practice Description

Automated dispensing systems are drug storage devices or cabinets that electronically dispense medications in a controlled fashion and track medication use. Their principal advantage lies in permitting nurses to obtain medications for inpatients at the point of use. Most systems require user identifiers and passwords, and internal electronic devices track nurses accessing the system, track the patients for whom medications are administered, and provide usage data to the hospital's financial office for the patients' bills.

These automated dispensing systems can be stocked by centralized or decentralized pharmacies. Centralized pharmacies prepare and distribute medications from a central location within the hospital. Decentralized pharmacies reside on nursing units or wards, with a single decentralized pharmacy often serving several units or wards. These decentralized pharmacies usually receive their medication stock and supplies from the hospital's central pharmacy.

More advanced systems provide additional information support aimed at enhancing patient safety through integration into other external systems, databases, and the Internet. Some models use machine-readable code for medication dispensing and administration. Three types of automated dispensing devices were analysed in the studies reviewed here, the McLaughlin dispensing system, the Baxter ATC-212 dispensing system, and the Pyxis Medstation Rx. Their attributes are described below.

- The McLaughlin dispensing system includes a bedside dispenser, a programmable magnetic card, and a pharmacy computer. It is a locked system that is loaded with the medications prescribed for a patient. At the appropriate dosing time, the bedside dispenser drawer unlocks automatically to allow a dose to be removed and administered. A light above the patient's door illuminates at the appropriate dosing time. Only certain medications fit in the compartmentalized cabinet (such as tablets, capsules, small pre-filled syringes, and ophthalmic drops).
- The Baxter ATC-212 dispensing system uses a microcomputer to pack unit-dose tablets and capsules for oral administration. It is usually installed at the pharmacy. Medications are stored in calibrated canisters that are designed specifically for each medication. Canisters are assigned a numbered location, which is thought to reduce mix-up errors upon dispensing. When an order is sent to the microcomputer, a tablet is dispensed from a particular canister. The drug is ejected into a strip-packing device where it is labeled and hermetically sealed.

— The Pyxis Medstation, Medstation Rx, and Medstation Rx 1000 are automated dispensing devices kept on the nursing unit. These machines are often compared to automatic teller machines (ATMs). The Medstation interfaces with the pharmacy computer. Physicians' orders are entered into the pharmacy computer and then transferred to the Medstation where patient profiles are displayed to the nurse who accesses the medications for verified orders. Each nurse is provided with a password that must be used to access the Medstation. Pharmacists or technicians keep these units loaded with medication. Charges are made automatically for drugs dispensed by the unit. Earlier models had sufficient memory to contain data for about one week, and newer models can store data for longer periods.

Studies reviewed did not include the automated dispensing systems manufactured by Omnicell, which produces point-of-use systems that can be integrated into a hospital's information system. Omnicell systems are also capable of being integrated into external support systems that support machine-readable code, drug information services, and medication error reporting systems.

Prevalence and Severity of the Target Safety Problem

Medication errors within hospitals occur with 2% to 17% of doses ordered for inpatients. It has been suggested that the rate of inpatient medication errors is one per patient per inpatient day. The specific medication errors targeted by automated dispensing systems are those related to drug dispensing and administration. Even with the use of unit-doses errors still occur at the dispensing and administration stages of the medication use process. For instance, in one large study of 530 medical errors in 10,070 written orders for drugs (5.3 errors/100 orders), pharmacy dispensing accounted for 11% of errors and nursing administration 38%.

Opportunities for Impact

Automated dispensing devices have become increasingly common either to supplement or replace unit-dose distribution systems in an attempt to improve medication availability, increase the efficiency of drug dispensing and billing, and reduce errors. A 1999 national survey of drug dispensing and administration practices indicated that 38% of responding hospitals used automated medication dispensing units and 8.2% used machine-readable coding with dispensing. Three-fourths of respondents stated that their pharmacy was centralized and of these centralized pharmacies, 77% were not automated. Hospitals with automated centralized pharmacies reported that greater than 50% of their inpatient doses were dispensed via centralized automated systems. Half of all responding hospitals used a decentralized medication storage system. One-third of hospitals with automated storage and dispensing systems were linked to the pharmacy computer. Importantly, about half of the surveyed hospitals reported drug distributions that bypassed the pharmacy including floor stock, borrowing patients' medications, and hidden drug supplies.

Study Designs

There were no true randomized trials. One crossover study of the McLaughlin dispensing system randomized nurses to work with the intervention medication system or the control system. We classified this as a Level 2 study, since, from the patient perspective, the design is that of a non-randomized trial. Other studies included in this review consisted of retrospective observational studies with before-after or cross-sectional design (Level 3). The reviewed studies described dispensing systems for orally administered medications, and were published between 1984 and 1995.

Study Outcomes

All studies measured rates of medication errors (Level 2 outcome). Four studies detected errors by direct observation using a methodology that was first described by Barker. Direct observation methods have been criticized because of purported Hawthorne effect (bias involving changed behaviour resulting from measurements requiring direct observation of study subjects). However, proponents of the method state that such effects are short-lived, dissipating within hours of observation. Dean and Barber have recently demonstrated the validity and reliability of direct observational methods to detect medication administration errors. Another study, a Level 3 design, determined errors by inspecting dispensed drugs.

Evidence for Effectiveness of the Practice

The evidence provided by the limited number of available, generally poor quality studies does not suggest that automated dispensing devices reduce medication errors. There is also no evidence to suggest that outcomes are improved with the use of these devices. Most of the published studies comparing automated devices with unit-dose dispensing systems report reductions in medication errors of omission and scheduling errors with the former. The studies suffer from multiple problems with confounding, as they often compare hospitals or nursing care units that may differ in important respects other than the medication distribution system.

Potential for Harm

Human intervention may prevent these systems from functioning as designed. Pharmacists and nurses can override some of the patient safety features. When the turn around time for order entry into the automated system is prolonged, nurses may override the system thereby defeating its purpose. Furthermore, the automated dispensing systems must be refilled intermittently to replenish exhausted supplies. Errors can occur during the course of refilling these units or medications may shift from one drawer or compartment to another causing medication mix-ups. Either of these situations can slip past the nurse at medication administration.

The results of the study of the McLaughlin dispensing system indicated that though overall errors were reduced compared to unit-dose (10.6% vs. 15.9%), errors decreased for 13 of 20 nurses but increased for the other 7 nurses. In a study of Medstation Rx vs. unit-dose, errors decreased in the cardiovascular surgery unit, where errors were recorded by work measurement observations. However, errors increased over 30% in 6 of 7 nurses after automated dispensing was installed in the cardiovascular intensive care unit, where incident reports and medication error reports were both used for ascertaining errors, raising the question of measurement bias. Finally, in a study primarily aimed at determining differences in errors for ward and unit-dose dispensing systems, a greater error prevalence was found for medications dispensed using Medstation Rx compared with those dispensed using unit-dose or non-automated floor stock (17.1% vs. 5.4%).

Costs and Implementation

The cost of automated dispensing mainly involves the capital investment of renting or purchasing equipment for dispensing, labeling, and tracking (which often is done by computer). A 1995 study revealed that the cost of Medstation Rx to cover 10 acute care units (330 total beds) and 4 critical care units (48 total beds) in a large referral hospital would be $1.28 million over 5 years. Taking into account costs saved from reduced personnel and decreased drug waste, the units had the potential to save $1 million over 5 years. Most studies that examine economic impact found a trade-off between reductions in medication dispensing time for pharmacy and medication administration time for nursing personnel. A common complaint by nurses is long waiting lines at Pyxis Medstations if there are not enough machines. Nurses must access these machines using a nurse-specific password. This limited access to drugs on nursing units decreases drug waste and pilferage.

Comment

Although the implementation of automated dispensing reduces personnel time for medication administration and improves billing efficiency, reduction in medication errors have not been uniformly realised. Indeed, some studies suggest that errors may increase with some forms of automation. The results of the study of the McLaughlin Dispensing System by Barker et al showed considerable nurse-to-nurse variability in the error rate between the automated system and conventional unit dose. Qualitative data aimed at determining the reason for this variability would be useful. The study by Klein et al indicated little difference in the accuracy of medication cart filling by the Baxter ATC-212 (0.65%) versus filling by technicians (0.84%). Borel and Rascati found that medication errors, largely those related to the time of administration, were fewer after implementation of the Pyxis Medstation Rx (10.4%) compared with the historical period (16.9%). These results are consistent with a more recent study by Shirley, that found a 31% increase in the on-time administration of scheduled doses after installation of the Medstation Rx 1000. In contrast, errors were greater after Medstation Rx in the study by Schwarz and Brodowy, increasing on 6 of 7 nursing units by more than 30%. Finally, Dean et al found half the errors in a ward-based system without automation in the United Kingdom (3.0%, 95% CI: 2.4-3.7%) compared with an automated unit-dose medication distribution system in the United States (6.9%, 95% CI: 5.2-8.5%).

The practical limitations of the systems were illustrated by a variety of process deviations observed by Borel and Rascati. These included nurses waiting at busy administration times, removal of doses ahead of time to circumvent waiting, and overriding the device when a dose was needed quickly. These procedural failures emphasize an often-raised point with the introduction of new technologies, namely that the latest innovations are not a solution for inadequate or faulty processes or procedures.

Although automated dispensing systems are increasingly common, it appears they may not be completely beneficial in their current form. Further study is needed to demonstrate the effectiveness of newer systems such as the Omnicell automated dispensing devices. If the standard, namely unit-dose dispensing, is to be improved, such improvements will likely derive from robotics and informatics. To document impact of automated dispensing devices on patient safety, studies are needed comparing unit-dose dispensing with automated dispensing devices. Until the benefits of automated dispensing devices become clearer, the opportunities for impact of these devices is uncertain.

THE CORRECT CODING INITIATIVE

History

In 1994, the Health Care Financing Administration (HCFA) awarded a contract to AdminaStar Federal, the Indiana Medicare carrier, to define correct coding practices that would serve as the basis for national Medicare. Based upon their review of CPT code descriptors, CPT coding instructions, review of existing and national coding edits and review of Medicare billing history, AdminaStar developed 94,000 questionable coding combinations. These combinations can be broken down into two main types: (1) comprehensive and component code combinations; and (2) mutually exclusive coding combinations that represent services or procedures that would not or could not be performed at the same time based on the CPT code description or standard medical practice.

The list of 94,000 coding combinations was distributed to the ACR and other specialty societies, as well as Medicare carrier medical directors for review and comment in December 1994. Based on these comments, AdminaStar revised the policy by removing 5,711 code combinations. Using the remaining coding combinations, AdminaStar developed a "code matrix" that automatically identifies inappropriate CPT code combinations and determines appropriate payment. This code matrix was implemented on Jan. 1, 1996. By implementing the coding matrix, Medicare was following a trend instituted by private payors. All private insurers, such as Blue Cross/Blue Shield and other indemnity insurers, use a code matrix to look for instances where procedures are inappropriately unbundled.

AdminaStar continues to provide additions to the Correct Coding Initiative. These are reviewed by the ACR and all other medical societies. Few, if any, of the additional code pairs added are used by rheumatologists.

In addition to the contract with AdminaStar, HCFA has purchased a coding edit programme from HBO and Co., a private medical software firm. Unlike the Correct Coding Initiative, the code pairs in this programme have not been reviewed by medical societies. Because the programme is proprietary, HCFA agreed not to make the edits public. The American Medical Association has worked with HCFA to gain the release of the philosophy behind the code edits, but restrictions still prevent specialty societies from reviewing this information. Many within organised medicine call these "black box edits" because they are developed and implemented in the dark.

Physicians will only learn which code pairs are prohibited in this "black box" programme when they receive payment denials. If a claim is rejected because services billed are not allowed on the same day, you should check the code pairs against the latest edition of the Correct Coding Initiative book. If the code pair is not present there, you have likely discovered one of the "black box" edits. You may request some explanation from the carrier, but it will likely be vague. The ACR is working with the AMA to protest the inclusion of "black box" edits.

How Correct Coding Policies Affect Rheumatology Coding

According to the Correct Coding policy, in order to submit a CPT code to Medicare, the provider must have performed all services included in the code descriptor. Otherwise, the provider must submit a less comprehensive code. Providers must not submit codes describing components of a comprehensive code in addition to the comprehensive code. Components are services necessary to accomplish the more comprehensive procedure/service. For example, when billing CPT code 20600 (Arthrocentesis, aspiration and/or injection; small joint, bursa or ganglion cyst), one should not also bill CPT code 20550 (Injection, tendon sheath, ligament, trigger points or ganglion cyst). CPT code 20600 is considered a "comprehensive procedure code." Other code bundles frequently encountered by rheumatologists include 20605/20550 and 20610/20550.

Coding Tips: How to Prevent Erroneous Denials

To prevent erroneous denials of claims for several procedures, HCFA developed the "-59" modifier to denote "a distinct procedural service." Modifier "-59" may be used to indicate that a procedure or service was distinct or separate from other services performed on the same day (i.e., different session or patient encounter, different procedure or surgery, different site, separate lesion or separate injury). For example, CPT codes 20605 and 20550 have been bundled. You should append the "-59" modifier on CPT code 20550 if you use both codes during a visit. The medical record should clearly reflect that a different procedure was performed or that the same procedure was performed on a different site. The "-59" modifier does not replace any existing modifiers. It is also important to note that, if an anatomic modifier (-LT, -RT, or digit modifiers) is available, use of this type of modifier is preferred over the application of modifier "-59."

If you do experience a claim denial that you feel is unjust based on this information, you should appeal the decision through the existing channels with your local Medicare carrier. Existing national Medicare payment policies are not changed by the new Correct Coding policy

The CPT Coding System

Physicians' Current Procedural Terminology (CPT) is a systematic listing and coding of services and procedures performed by physicians. The CPT system provides a uniform language for communication with third-party payors for reimbursement purposes. CPT codes are also used to record the services rendered to an individual patient and are compiled by third-party payors and government agencies as a record of an individual physician's activities.

CPT codes consist of five-digit numbers that represent individual services and procedures. They are divided into six major categories: Evaluation and Management (E/M), Anesthesiology, Surgery, Radiology, Pathology, Laboratory, and Medicine. These codes may be further defined by starred (*) designations for certain minor surgical procedures, and by modifiers to help explain an unusual circumstance associated with a service or procedure.

The American Medical Association (AMA) publishes the CPT codes on a yearly basis. All CPT five-digit numeric codes, descriptions, numeric modifiers, instructions, guidelines, and other material are Copyright 1998, American Medical Association. All rights reserved. *Note: Just because a CPT code exists does not mean that all insurers reimburse for it.*

Codes for needle muscle biopsy and injection of tendons and various joints and bursae are in the surgical section under the musculoskeletal section. Codes for interpretation of radiographs and laboratory tests are found in the radiology and laboratory code sections, respectively.

Physicians should read the coding guidelines published in this manual and the AMA CPT manual very carefully. In addition, Appendix B of the AMA CPT manual should be referenced for additional code changes, deletions and additions.

Definitions

Certain key words and phrases are used throughout the E/M section of the AMA CPT manual. The following definitions from the AMA CPT manual are intended to reduce the potential for differing interpretations and to increase the consistency of reporting physicians in differing specialties.

New and Established Patient

A *new patient* is one who has not received any professional services from the physician or another physician of the same specialty who belongs to the same group practice, within the past three years.

An *established patient* is one who has received professional services from the physician or another physician of the same specialty who belongs to the same group practice within the past three years.

In the instance where a physician is on call for or covering for another physician, the patient's encounter will be classified as it would have been by the physician who is not available.

No distinction is made between new and established patients in the emergency department. E/M services in the emergency department category may be reported for any new or established patient who presents for treatment in the emergency department.

Consultation

A *consultation* is a type of service provided by a physician whose opinion or advice regarding evaluation and management of a specific problem is requested by another physician or other appropriate source. A physician consultant may initiate diagnostic and/or therapeutic services.

If a consultant subsequently assumes responsibility for management of a portion or all of the patient's condition, the consultation codes should not be used. The established patient office visit codes must be used for follow-up visits. Four categories of consultations are recognized: office, initial inpatient, follow-up inpatient and confirmatory.

Concurrent Care

Concurrent care is the provision of similar services, (e.g., hospital visits) to the same patient by more than one physician on the same day. When concurrent care is provided, no special reporting is required.

Chief Complaint

The *chief complaint* is a concise statement describing the symptom, problem, condition, diagnosis or other factor that is the reason for the encounter, usually stated in the patient's words.

History of Present Illness

The *history of present illness* refers to the chronological description of the development of the patient's present illness from the first sign and/or symptom to the present. This includes a description of location, quality, severity, timing, context, modifying factors and associated signs and symptoms significantly related to the presenting problem(s).

System Review (Review of Systems)

An inventory of body systems obtained through a series of questions seeking to identify signs and/or symptoms which the patient may be experiencing or has experienced. The review of systems helps define the problem, clarify the differential diagnoses, identify needed testing or serves as baseline data on other systems that might be affected by any possible management options. For the purposes of CPT the following elements of a system review have been identified:

— Constitutional symptoms (fever, weight loss, etc.)
— Eyes
— Ears, nose, mouth, throat
— Cardiovascular
— Respiratory
— Gastrointestinal
— Genitourinary

— Musculoskeletal
— Integumentary (skin and/or breast)
— Neurological
— Psychiatric
— Endocrine
— Hematologic/Lymphatic
— Allergic/Immunologic

Past History

A review of the patient's past experiences with illnesses, injuries and treatments that includes significant information about:

— Prior major illnesses and injuries
— Prior operations
— Prior hospitalisations
— Current medications
— Allergies (e.g., drug, food)
— Age-appropriate immunisation status
— Age-appropriate feeding/dietary status

Family History

A review of medical events in the patient's family that includes significant information about:

— The health status or cause of death of parents, siblings and children
— Specific diseases related to problems identified in the Chief Complaint or History of the

Present Illness and/or System Review

— Diseases of family members which may be hereditary or place the patient at risk

Social History

An age appropriate review of past and current activities that includes significant information about:

— Marital status and/or living arrangements

— Current employment

— Occupational history

— Use of drugs, alcohol and tobacco

— Level of education

— Sexual history

— Other relevant social factors

Levels of Evaluation and Management Services

Seven components are recognized as descriptors for the levels of Evaluation and Management (E/M) services, six of which are used in defining the levels of E/M services. These components are: *history, examination, medical decision making, counseling, coordination of care, nature of the presenting problem, and time.* The first three of these components (history, examination and medical decision making) are considered the *key* factors in selecting a level of E/M service. The next three factors (counseling, coordination of care and the nature of the presenting problem) are considered *contributory* factors in choosing an E/M service for the majority of encounters. The final component — time — is predominantly included to assist the physician and is considered a key component only if counseling/coordination of care composed more than 50 percent of the physician-patient face-to-face encounter.

The actual performance and/or interpretation of diagnostic tests and studies ordered during a patient encounter may have its own CPT code, and these codes may be reported separately in addition to the appropriate E/M code.

For some studies, the performance of the study can be separated from the interpretation. For example, if a physician refers a patient to a radiology center for the technical portion of a DEXA scan but asks that the raw data be sent back for interpretation, the physician would bill only for the professional component of the test by using the appropriate CPT code with the modifier "-26" appended.

In some cases, it may be possible to bill for interpretation of diagnostic tests or studies even if they have been previously interpreted by another physician. A separately identifiable report written by the physician re-reviewing the results is necessary. Use the modifier "-26" to indicate that only the professional component was performed. Medicare carriers generally will not pay for multiple interpretations of x-rays or lab tests because they consider this review to be a necessary part of medical decision making for evaluation and management codes.

History: The extent of the history is dependent upon clinical judgment and on the nature of the presenting problem(s). The levels of E/M services recognize four types of history that are defined as follows:

Problem Focused: chief complaint; brief history of present illness or problem

Expanded Problem Focused: chief complaint; brief history of present illness; problem pertinent system review

Detailed: chief complaint; extended history of present illness; problem pertinent system review extended to include a review of a limited number of additional systems; pertinent past, family, and/or social history directly related to the patient's problems

Comprehensive: chief complaint; extended history of present illness; review of systems that is directly related to the problem(s) identified in the history of the present illness plus a review of all additional body systems; complete past, family and social history

Examination: The extent of the examination performed is dependent on clinical judgment and on the nature of the presenting problem(s). The levels of E/M services recognize four types of examination that are defined as follows:

Problem Focused: a limited examination of the affected body area or organ system

Expanded Problem Focused: a limited examination of the affected body area or organ system and other symptomatic or related organ system(s)

Detailed: an extended examination of the affected body area(s) and other symptomatic or related organ system(s)

Comprehensive: a general multi-system examination or a complete examination of a single organ system

For the purposes of these CPT definitions, the following *body areas* are recognized:

— Head, including the face
— Neck
— Chest, including breasts and axilla
— Abdomen
— Genitalia, groin, buttocks
— Back
— Each extremity

For the purposes of these CPT definitions, the following organ systems are recognized:

— Eyes

- Ears, Nose, Mouth and Throat
- Cardiovascular
- Respiratory
- Gastrointestinal
- Genitourinary
- Musculoskeletal
- Skin
- Neurologic
- Psychiatric
- Hematologic/Lymphatic/Immunologic
- Hematologic/Lymphatic/Immunologic

Medical Decision Making: Medical decision making refers to the complexity of establishing a diagnosis and/or selecting a management option as measured by:

- The number of possible diagnoses and/or the number of management options that must be considered
- The amount and/or complexity of medical records, diagnostic tests and/or other information that must be obtained, reviewed and analysed
- The risk of significant complications, morbidity and/or mortality, as well as comorbidities, associated with the patient's presenting problem(s), the diagnostic procedure(s) and/or the possible management options

Four types of medical decision making are recognized: *straightforward, low complexity, moderate complexity,* and *high complexity*. To qualify for a given type of decision making, two of the three elements in the following table must be met or exceeded:

Counseling: Counseling is a discussion with a patient and/or family concerning one or more of the following areas:

— Diagnostic results, impressions and/or recommended diagnostic studies

— Prognosis

— Risks and benefits of management (treatment) options

— Instructions for management (treatment) and/or follow-up

— Importance of compliance with chosen management (treatment) options

— Risk factor reduction

— Patient and family education

Under Medicare, family counseling cannot be credited toward "counseling" in an evaluation and management code in the office unless the patient is present. The counseling must deal with the patient's problems, not the family's difficulty in handling the patient.

Coordination of Care: In the case where counseling and/or coordination of care composes more than 50 percent of the physician-patient and/or physician-family encounter (face-to-face time in the office or other outpatient setting or floor/unit time in the hospital or nursing facility), time is considered the key or controlling factor to qualify for a particular level of E/M service. The extent of counseling and/or coordination of care must be documented in the medical record. You may also want to indicate the time involved and a brief outline of the issues discussed.

Nature of Presenting Problem: A presenting problem is a disease, condition, illness, injury, symptom, sign, finding, complaint or other reason for encounter, with or without a diagnosis being established at the time of the encounter. The E/M codes recognize five types of presenting problems that are defined as follows:

Minimal: A problem that may not require the presence of the physician, but service is provided under the physician's supervision

Self-limited or Minor: A problem that runs a definite and prescribed course, is transient in nature and is not likely to permanently alter health status OR has a good prognosis with management/compliance

Low severity: A problem where the risk of morbidity without treatment is low; there is little to no risk of mortality without treatment; full recovery without functional impairment is expected

Moderate severity: A problem where the risk of morbidity without treatment is moderate; there is moderate risk of mortality without treatment; uncertain prognosis OR increased probability of prolonged functional impairment

High severity: A problem where the risk of morbidity without treatment is high to extreme; there is a moderate to high risk or mortality without treatment OR high probability of severe, prolonged functional impairment.

Time: The inclusion of time as an explicit factor is done only to assist physicians in selecting the most appropriate levels of E/M services. It should be recognized that the specific times expressed in the visit code descriptors are averages and, therefore, represent a range of times which may be higher or lower depending on actual clinical circumstances.

Intra-service times are defined as *face-to-face* time for office and other outpatient visits and as *unit / floor* time for hospital and other inpatient visits. This distinction is necessary because most of the work of typical office visits takes place during the face-to-face time with the patient, while most of the work of typical hospital visits takes place during the time spent on the patient's floor or unit.

Modifiers

Modifiers may be used to inform the payor that:

— A service or procedure has been increased or reduced

— Only part of a service was performed

— A bilateral procedure was performed

— An adjunctive service was performed

— A service or procedure has both a professional and a technical component

— A service or procedure was performed more than once

— A service or procedure was performed by more than one physician and/or in more than one location

— Unusual events occurred.

A modifier provides the means by which a physician can communicate to payors that a specific service or procedure was performed, but due to certain circumstances the service provided was different from that which the CPT code normally identifies. This is meant to justify a claim for services that are different from usual. What is most significant, however, is the fact that the service has not been changed in its definition or code.

A modifier is identified in either of two ways. The modifier may be reported by a two-digit number placed after the usual procedure number from which it is separated by a hyphen. Or, the modifier may be reported by a separate five-digit code that is used in addition to the procedure code. (In the case of modifiers "-24" and "-25," the two digit number or five digit code is reported after the appropriate level of E/M service.) Modifiers most likely to be used by rheumatologists are as follows:

-21 Prolonged Evaluation and Management Services. When the face-to-face or floor/unit service(s) provided is prolonged or otherwise greater than that usually required for the highest level of evaluation and management service within a given category, it may be identified by adding modifier "-21" to the evaluation and management code number or by use of the separate five-digit modifier code 09921. *Note: HCFA allows reimbursement for prolonged services codes (99354-99357) rather than modifier "-21." The prolonged service codes may only be used with certain E/M codes. For instance, 99354 (face-to-face prolonged care in outpatient setting, first hour) may only be used in conjunction with 99201-99215, 99241-99245 and 99301-99350.*

-24 Unrelated Evaluation and Management Service by the Same Physician During a Postoperative Period. The physician may need to indicate that an evaluation and management service was performed during a postoperative period for a reason(s) unrelated to the original procedure. This circumstance may be reported by adding the modifier "-24" to the appropriate level of E/M service code, or by use of the separate five-digit modifier 09924 in addition to coding for the procedure.

-25 Significant, Separately Identifiable Evaluation and Management Service by the Same Physician on the Same Day of the Procedure or Other Service. The physician may need to indicate that on the day a procedure or service identified by a CPT code was performed, the patient's condition required a significant, separately identifiable E/M service above and beyond the other service provided or beyond the usual preoperative and postoperative care associated with the procedure that was performed. This circumstance may be reported by adding the modifier "-25" to the appropriate level of E/M service code or the separate five-digit modifier 09925 may be used. *Note: This modifier is not used to report an E/M service that results in a decision to perform surgery.*

-26 Professional Component. Certain procedures are a combination of a physician component and a technical component. When the physician component is reported separately, the service may be identified by adding the modifier "-26" to the usual procedure number or the service may be reported by use of the five-digit modifier code 09926.

-32 Mandated Services. Services related to mandated consultation and/or related services (e.g., PRO, third party payor) may be identified by adding the modifier "-32" to the basic procedure or the service may be reported by use of the five-digit modifier 09932.

-50 Bilateral Procedure. Unless otherwise identified in the listings, bilateral procedures that are performed at the same operative session should be identified by the appropriate five-digit code describing the first procedure. The five-digit procedure code should be followed by the modifier.

-51 Multiple Procedures. When multiple procedures, other than evaluation and management services, are performed on the same day or at the same session by the same provider, the primary procedure or service may be reported as listed. The additional, or lesser procedure(s) or service(s) may be identified by adding the modifier "-51" to the additional procedure or service code(s) or by use of the separate five-digit modifier 09951. *Note: This modifier may be used to report multiple medical procedures performed at the same session as well as a combination of medical and surgical procedures or several surgical procedures performed at the same operative session.*

-52 Reduced Services. Under certain circumstances, a service or procedure is partially reduced or eliminated at the physician's election. The service provided can be identified by its usual procedure number and the addition of the modifier "-52" signifying that the service is reduced. This provides a means of reporting reduced services without disturbing the identification of the basic service. Modifier code 09952 may be used as an alternative to modifier "-52."

-57 Decision for Surgery. An evaluation and management service that resulted in the initial decision to perform the surgery may be identified by adding the modifier "-57" to the appropriate level of E/M service, or the separate five-digit modifier 09957 may be used. (This applies to major surgical procedures with 90 global days, not to minor surgical procedures like arthrocentesis.)

-59 Distinct Procedural Service. Under certain circumstances, the physician may need to indicate that a procedure or service was distinct or independent from other services performed on the same day. Modifier "-59" is used to identify procedures/services that are not normally reported together, but are appropriate under the circumstances. This may represent a different session or patient encounter, different procedure or surgery, different site or organ system, separate incision/excision, separate lesion or separate injury (or area of injury in extensive injuries) not ordinarily encountered or performed on the same day by the same physician. However, when another already established modifier is appropriate it should be used rather than modifier "-59." Only if no more descriptive modifier is available, and the use of modifier "-59" best explains the circumstances, should modifier "-59" be used. Modifier code 09959 may be used as an alternative to modifier "59."

-76 Repeat Procedure by Same Physician. The physician may need to indicate that a procedure or service was repeated subsequent to the original service. This circumstance may be reported by adding the modifier "-76" to the repeated service, or the separate five-digit modifier code 09976 may be used.

-77 Repeat Procedure by Another Physician. The physician may need to indicate that a basic procedure performed by another physician had to be repeated. This situation may be reported by adding modifier "-77" to the repeated service, or the separate five digit-modifier code 09977 may be used.

-78 Return to the Operating Room for a Related Procedure During the Postoperative Period. The physician may need to indicate that another procedure was performed during the postoperative period of the initial procedure. When this subsequent procedure is related to the first and requires the use of the operating room it may be reported by adding the modifier "-78" to the related procedure or by using the separate five-digit modifier 09978. *Note: For repeat procedures on the same day, see modifier "-76."*

-79 Unrelated Procedure or Service by the Same Physician During the Postoperative Period. The physician may need to indicate that the performance of a procedure or service during the postoperative period was unrelated to the original procedure. This circumstance may be reported by using the modifier "-79" or by using the separate five-digit modifier 09979. *Note: For repeat procedures on the same day, see modifier "-76."*

2

Health and Medical Informatics and Services

INTRODUCTION TO HEALTH INFORMATICS: THE SYSTEMS SCIENCE OF HEALTH CARE

If physiology literally means 'the logic of life', and pathology is 'the logic of disease', then health informatics is the logic of healthcare. It is the rational study of the way we think about patients, and the way that treatments are defined, selected and evolved. It is the study of how clinical knowledge is created, shaped, shared and applied. Ultimately, it is the study of how we organise ourselves to create and run healthcare organisations. With such a pivotal role, it is likely that in the next century, the study of informatics will become as fundamental to the practice of medicine as anatomy has been to the last.

Health informatics is thus as much about computers as cardiology is about stethoscopes. Rather than drugs, X-ray machines or surgical instruments, the tools of informatics are more likely to be clinical guidelines, formal health languages, information systems, or communication systems like the Internet. These tools, however, are only a means to an end, which is the delivery of the best possible healthcare.

Although the name 'health informatics' only came into use around 1973 (Protti, 1995), it is a study that is as old as healthcare itself. It was born the day that a clinician first wrote down some impressions about a patient's illness, and used these to learn how to treat their next patient. Informatics has grown considerably as a clinical discipline in recent years fuelled, in part no doubt, by the advances in computer technology. What has fundamentally changed is our ability to describe and manipulate health knowledge at a highly abstract level, as has our ability to build up rich communication systems to support the process of healthcare.

We can formally say that health informatics is the study of information and communication systems in healthcare. Health informatics is particularly focused on:

1. Understanding the fundamental nature of these information and communication systems, and describing the principles which shape them,
2. Developing interventions which can improve upon existing information and communication systems,
3. Developing methods and principles which allow such interventions to be designed,
4. Evaluating the impact of these interventions on the way individuals or organisations work, or on the outcome of the work.

Specific subspecialties of health informatics include clinical informatics, which focuses on the use of information in support of patient care and bioinformatics, which focuses on the use of genomic and other biological information.

The Rise of Health Informatics

Perhaps the greatest change in clinical thinking over the last two centuries has been the ascendancy of the scientific method. Since its acceptance, it has become the lens through which we see the world, and governs everything from the way we view disease, through to the way we battle it. It is now hard to imagine just how controversial the introduction of theory and experimental method into medicine once was. Then, it was strongly opposed by the views of the empiricists, who believed that observation, rather than theoretical conjecture, was the only basis for the rational practice of medicine. With this perspective, it is almost uncanny to hear again the old empiricists' argument that 'healthcare is an art', and not a place for unnecessary speculation or formalisation. This time, the empiricists are fighting against those who wish to develop formal theoretical methods to regulate the communal practice of healthcare. Words like quality and safety, clinical audit, outcome measures, healthcare rationing and evidence-based practice now define the new intellectual battleground. While the advance of science pushes clinical knowledge down to a fine-grained molecular and genetic level, it is events at the other end of the scale are forcing us to change. Firstly, the enterprise of healthcare has become so large that it now consumes more national resources than any country is willing to bear. Despite sometimes heroic efforts to control this growth in consumption, the healthcare budget continues to expand. There is thus a social and economic imperative to control healthcare and minimise its drain on social resources. The structure of clinical practice is also coming under pressure from within.

The scientific method, long the backbone of medicine, is now in some ways under threat. The reason for this is not that experimental science is unable to answer our questions about the nature of disease and its treatment. Rather, it is almost too good at its job. As clinical research ploughs ahead in laboratories and clinics across the world, like some great information machine, health practitioners are being swamped by its results. So much research is now published each week that it can literally take decades for the results of clinical trials to translate into changes in clinical practice. So, healthcare workers find themselves practising with ever restricting resources and unable, even if they had the time, to keep abreast of the knowledge of best practice hidden in the literature. As a consequence, the scientific basis of clinical practice trails far behind that of clinical research. Two hundred years ago, enlightened physicians understood that empiricism needed to be replaced by a more formal and testable way of characterising disease and its treatment. The tool they used then was the scientific method. Today we are in analogous situation. Now the demand is that we replace the organisational processes and structures that force the arbitrary selection amongst treatments with ones that can be formalised, tested, and applied rationally. Modern healthcare has moved away from seeing disease in isolation, to understanding that illness occurs at a complex system level. Infection is not simply the result of the invasion of a pathogenic organism, but the complex interaction of an individual's immune system, nutritional status, environmental and genetic endowments.

By seeing things at a system level, we come ever closer to understanding what it really means to be diseased, and how that state can be reversed. We now need to make the same conceptual leap and begin to see the great systems of knowledge that enmesh the delivery of healthcare. These systems produce our knowledge, tools, languages and methods. Thus, a new treatment is never created and tested in intellectual isolation. It gains significance as part of a greater system of knowledge, since it occurs in the context of previous treatments and insights, as well as the context of a society's resources and needs. Further, the work does not finish when we scientifically prove a treatment works. We must try to communicate this new knowledge and help others to understand, apply, and adapt it.

These then are the challenges for healthcare. Can we put together rational structures for the way clinical evidence is pooled, communicated and applied to routine care? Can we develop organisational processes and structures that minimise the resources we use and maximise the benefits delivered? And finally, what tools and methods need to be developed to help achieve these aims in a manner that is practicable, testable and in keeping with the fundamental goal of healthcare - the relief from disease? The role of health informatics is to develop a systems science for healthcare that provides a rational basis to answer these questions, as well as to create the tools to achieve these goals. The scope of informatics is thus enormous. It finds application in the design of clinical decision support systems for practitioners, in the development of computer tools for research, and in the study of the very essence of medicine - its corpus of knowledge. Yet the modern discipline of health informatics is still relatively young.

Many different groups within healthcare are addressing the issues raised here and not always in a co-ordinated fashion. Indeed, these groups are not always even aware that their efforts are connected, nor that their concerns are ones of informatics. The first goal of this book is to present a unifying set of basic informatics principles which influence everything from the delivery of care to an individual patient through to the design of whole healthcare systems. Its next goal is to present the breadth of issues which concern informatics, show how they are related, and to encourage research into understanding the common principles that connect them. Each area that is covered has been written with three criteria in mind - its possibility, its practicability, and its desirability. Possibility reflects the science of informatics - what in theory can be achieved? Practicability addresses the potential for successfully engineering a system or introducing a new process - what can actually be done given the constraints of the real world? Desirability looks at the fundamental motivation for using a given process or technology. These criteria are suggested in part because we need to evolve a framework to judge the claims made for new technologies and those who seek to profit from them. Just as there is a long-standing symbiosis between the pharmaceutical industry and medicine, there is a newer and consequently less examined relationship between healthcare and the computing and telecommunication industries. Clinicians should try to judge the claims of these newcomers in the same cautious way that they would examine claims about a new drug (Wyatt, 1987) and perhaps more so, given that clinicians are far more knowledgeable about pharmacology than they are about informatics and telecommunications.

Overview of the Book

The book is organised into a number of parts, all of which revolve around the two distinct strands of information and communication. While the unique character of each strand is explored individually, there is also an emphasis on understanding the rich way in which they can interact and complement each other.

Part 1 - Basic Concepts in Informatics

Like healthcare, informatics has both theoretical and applied aspects to its study. This first part of the book is focused on developing an intuitive understanding of the basic theoretical concepts needed to approach informatics practice in a principled way. Three fundamental ideas underpin the study of informatics - the notions of what constitutes a model, what one means by information, and what defines a system. Each of these three ideas is explored to develop an understanding of the nature of information and communication systems. A recurring theme in this part will be the need to understand the limitations imposed upon us whenever we create or use a model of the world. Understanding these limitations defines the ultimate limits of possibility for informatics, irrespective of whichever technology one may wish to apply in its service.

Part 2 – Informatics Skills

Building upon the concepts in Part one, the second part of the book looks at the practical lessons that can be drawn from informatics to guide everyday clinical activity. Every clinical action, every treatment choice and investigation, is shaped by the available information and how effectively that information is communicated. Five basic clinical informatics skills are explored, each with their own individual chapter:

1. Communicating effectively is based upon understanding cognitive models of information processing, and is constantly challenged by the limits of human attention, and the imperfection of models;
2. Structuring information, with a particular focus on the patient record, is shown to be dependent upon the task at hand, the channel used to communicate the message, and the agent who will receive the message;
3. Questioning others to find information is essential in clinical practice to fill the ever present gaps in every individual's knowledge;
4. Searching for knowledge describes the broader strategic process of knowing where to ask questions, evaluating answers, and refining questions in the light of previous actions, and occurs in many different settings, from when patient's are interviewed and

examined, through to when treatment options are canvassed;

5. Making Decisions occurs when all the available information needed has been assembled using the other informatics skills, and attempts to come up with the best alternative to solve a problem like selecting a treatment, based both upon the evidence from science, as well as the wishes and needs of individuals.

Part 3 - Information Systems in Healthcare

The chapters in this part explore the special character of information systems in healthcare. The clinical record is given many names and is discussed in many different guises throughout the book, and its role and scope are introduced here. Information systems like the electronic medical record are shown to manage a wide variety of activities. Ultimately, the way that these activities are modelled, measured and then managed is determined by information system design.

Sometimes, leaving things unsaid or informal is more productive than encoding them in a formal computer system. Consequently, the important concept of system formality is also introduced here, since it is not always appropriate to build information systems. Indeed it can often be counterproductive. Understanding the role of formality helps principled decisions to be made before information systems are introduced. The concept of formality also helps us to understand the different roles that communication and information systems play in healthcare. The final chapter in this part spends some time describing how one sets out to build such systems, and some of the design problems that bedevil that process.

Having laid down these foundational ideas in the first two parts of the book, the next two parts turn to focus on two information problems that are specific to healthcare - protocol-based care, and clinical coding.

Part 4 - Protocol-based Systems

Clinical guidelines or protocols have been in limited use for many years. The current emphasis on evidence-based clinical practice has made it more likely that healthcare workers will use, and perhaps be involved in the design and maintenance of protocols. In this part, the various forms and uses of protocols are introduced. The various roles that computer-based protocol systems can play in clinical practice are outlined. These cover both traditional 'passive' support where protocols are kept as a reference, and active systems in which the computer uses the protocol to assist in the delivery of care. For example, protocols incorporated into the electronic record can generate clinical alerts or make treatment recommendations. Their characteristic advantages and limitations of are also discussed and these are then used to formulate a set of protocol design principles.

Part 5 - Language, Coding and Classification in Healthcare

If the data contained in electronic patient record systems is to be analysed, then it needs to be accessible in some regular way. This is usually thwarted by the variations in health terminology used by different individuals, institutions and nations. To remedy the problem, large dictionaries of standardised clinical terms have been created.

The chapters in this section introduce the basic ideas of concepts, terms, codes and classifications, and demonstrate their various uses. The inherent advantages and limitations of using terms and codes are discussed. The last chapter in particular looks at some more advanced issues in coding, describing the theoretical limitations to coding, and outlines practical approaches to managing these issues, as well as presenting open research questions.

Part 6 - Communication Systems in Healthcare

While interpersonal communication skills are fundamental to patient care, the process of communication has, for a long time, not been well supported technologically. Now, with the widespread availability of communication systems supporting mobility, voice mail, electronic mail and video-conferencing, new possibilities arise. The chapters in this section introduce the basic types of communication services and explain the different benefits of each.

Given that much of the technology is new for many, one chapter is devoted to describing the basics of the various different communication systems now available. The final chapter in this part examines clinical communication and the field of telemedicine in the context of these new technologies. The potential of telemedical systems within different areas of healthcare is described, but the importance of carefully choosing the right set of technologies for a given problem is emphasised.

Part 7 - The Internet

Information systems are starting to become indistinguishable from communication ones, and this convergence is perhaps nowhere more apparent than with the Internet. This part explores in detail the phenomenal rise of the Internet and the World Wide Web, and examines why its technologies have proven to be so revolutionary. The complex way that the Web alters the balance of information publishing and access is explained, along with the consequences of these changes. The full impact of the Internet on healthcare has yet to be felt. Some of the many different ways that it will change healthcare are presented here, from the way communication occurs, through to the change it will have upon the doctor-patient relationship.

Part 8 - Intelligent Clinical Decision Support

The concluding chapters of the book look to some of the most complex computer systems created so far - those based upon the technologies of artificial intelligence (AI). The early promise of computer programmes that could assist clinicians in the process of diagnosis have come to fruition, and they are now in routine use in many clinical situations. AI techniques also permit the creation of systems able to assist with therapy planning, information seeking, and the generation of alerts.

The final chapters in this part look in detail at some of the specialised ways that decision technologies are applied in clinical practice. They find application in creating intelligent patient monitors, and potentially, autonomous therapeutic devices like self-adjusting patient ventilators. Along with communication technologies, they are essential components of biosurveillance systems. Finally, in the field of bioinformatics, human genome knowledge is harnessed using computer techniques, and reframes many classes of clinical decision as questions of genetics as much as pragmatic clinical science.

The Major Groups of People in Medical Informatic Ethics

- Health Care Professionals
- Applied Computing Professionals
- Scientists, Researchers
- Government Agencies
- Healthcare Product and Service Manufacturers, Online Medical Entrepreneurs
- Patients, Consumers

— Insurance Companies, Healthcare Management Organisations
— Administrators, Managers
— Medical Ethicists

Medicine, Ethics, & Medical Informatics

Trying to determine the scope of Ethics and Medical Informatics is much like the poem of "The Blind Men And The Elephant," where six blind men are each asked to describe an elephant. The descriptions of the elephant differed depending on which part of the animal was being viewed e.g. side, tusk, knee, ear, trunk, or tail. Each man, after experiencing the elephant, is convinced that his opinion was the only correct one. The field of Medical Informatics Ethics is a merger of several different areas of study. How it is described depends on who is viewing or experiencing the field. This field is even more confusing that the elephant. In our review we determined there are at least nine major groups of people involved, each of them with several subdivisions. Many of these groups have different, and at times conflicting, motivators for dealing with Medical Informatic Ethics. When possible in discussing the different components of Medical Informatics Ethics, we have included at least two of the areas involved e.g. medicine & ethics, computers & ethics, research & ethics.

Selecting the Topics

With so many different groups involved and so many areas of study, determining what topics to include in this Web Resource on Medicine, Ethics and Medical Informatics was quite a challenge. We started with the lecture topics for this seminar course from Christiansen on "Protecting personal health information in the Internet age" and Dr. Lundberg on "Electronic publishing in the Internet age."

We also reviewed course descriptions for Medical Informatics Ethics courses at OHSU and the Medical College of Wisconsin . The "Ethics and Health Informatics: Users, Standards, and Outcomes" chapter from the MINF 510 Text book by Goodman and Miller helped to identify their views of the major issues in medical informatics.

Our own interest in this topic had been demonstrated by the choice of term paper topics selected for other MINF courses. For the 512 course in Clinical Systems Ella's paper was an overview on smart cards that included a section on security and confidentiality. For the 510 Introduction of Medical Informatics course Kirsti's paper was on in the emerging field of Medical Internet Ethics. Additionally we posed the question to our MINF 528 classmates on this course's discussion board for input prior to creating this Web Resource.

Topics included in Ethics in Medical Informatics (MI-13201) Medical College of Wisconsin

- Privacy
- Security
- Confidentiality
- Encryption
- Coding
- Reimbursement
- Conflicts of Interest
- Reporting
- Protecting Information

Major Ethical Issues in Medical Informatics

- Confidentiality of electronically stored patient information.
- Appropriate selection and use of informatics tools in clinical settings.
- The determination of whom should use such tools.
- The role of system evaluation.

— The obligation of system developers, maintainers and vendors.

— The use of computers to track clinical outcomes to guide future practice.

— Informatics engenders many important legal and regulatory questions.

Ethics Courses – Descriptions

Topics included in MINF 515: Ethical and Legal Issues in Medical Informatics, OHSU

— The protection of confidentiality and privacy in an electronic environment

— Implications of the use of telemedicine and decision-support tools in diagnosis and treatment

— The implications of electronic communication for the physician-patient relationship

— Principles for design and functionality of consumer-oriented Web sites

Topics Selected for this Web Resource/Site Map

This web resource includes information and definitions for the areas of study involved in the Medical Informatics ethics. Additionally background information about each of the topics selected including resources, online when available is included. Finally some of the challenges facing the field of Medical Informatics Ethics are posed in the conclusions.

This resource is arranged in the following topics:

— Areas of Study

— The Scope of Medical Informatics Ethics

— The Legitimate Practitioners

— The Not-so Legitimate Practitioners

— Cybercrimes & Medicine
— Definitions: Ethical & Medical Informatics
— Ethics vs. Law
— Definitions
— Medical Ethics
— Medical Informatics
— Health/Healthcare Informatics/e-Health
— Telemedicine
— Medical Internet
— Scientific/Research Ethics
— Healthcare Ethics
— Clinical Ethics
— Computer Ethics
— Bioethics
— Medical Informatics Ethics
— Medical Internet Ethics
— Electronic Medical Records (EMR's)
— What are Electronic Medical Records?
— Who owns EMR's?
— How secure are EMR's?
— Medical records on smart cards
— Resources
— Privacy & Security/Protecting Patient Data
— Unique identifiers
— Electronic Mail
— Related Articles
— Resources

— Standardisation & HIPAA
— The Need for Standardisation in Health Informatics
— HIPAA: Health Insurance Portability and Accountability Act of 1996
— Background - HIPAA 1996
— Groups Pro and Con
— HIPAA - August 11, 1998
— HIPAA - December 20, 2000 - Clinton Administration
— HIPAA February 2001 - Bush Administration
— New HHS Secretary Issues New HIPAA Comment Period
— HIPAA and Informed Consent
— Resources
— Artificial Intelligence
— Artificial Intelligence in Medicine (AIM)
— Determining Appropriate Use & Users of Decision Support Systems
— Problems Encountered when using Clinical Computer Programmes for Policy or Practice
— 10 Criteria for System Scrutiny
— Future of Artificial Intelligence in Medicine
— Resources
— Science
— Medical Informatics, Science & Medicine
— A Hippocratic Oath for Scientists
— Hippocratic Oath for Scientists, Engineers and Executives
— A Graduate Pledge of Social and Environmental Responsibility

- An Oath for Computer Scientists?
- Other On-Line Science Ethics Resources
- Telemedicine
- Telemedicine
- Telepharmacy
- Resources and Organisations
- Projects and Services
- Related Articles
- Research
- Professional Integrity and Clinical Research
- What Makes Clinical Research Ethical?
- Informed Consent
- Ethical Considerations for Research and the Internet
- Establishing Ethical Standards for Internet Research
- A New Medium for Study - The Internet as a research arena for data collection

Conducting Ethical Research in Cyberspace

- Which Research Techniques work in Cyberspace?
- Real Life Example - Research & the Journey of Hearts Website
- Informed Consent and the Internet
- Increasing Connectivity - Internet as a Way to Get the Word out About Clinical Trials
- Marketing/Broadcasting - Using the Internet to solicit Research Subjects
- Resources
- Medical Internet
- Determining the Doctor/Patient, Provider/Client Relationship

— e-mail guidelines
— Online Medical Publishing
— Cyberplagerism
— Copyright - Poetry, Writing, Web-art, Graphics
— Guidelines for Rating Websites
— e-commerce, e-health
— Conclusions
— References
— Medical Informatics Ethics
— Medical Ethics
— Electronic Medical Records
— Privacy & Security
— Standardisation & HIPAA
— Artificial Intelligence
— Science & Ethics
— Telemedicine
— Research & Ethics
— Medical Internet
— Organisations
— Medical Informatics
— Informatic Standards Organisations
— HIPAA Organisations
— Artificial Intelligence
— Science & Ethics
— Telemedicine
— Research & Ethics
— Medical Online Publishing
— Medical Internet
— Patient Advocacy Groups/Privacy

MEDICAL INFORMATICS

Medical informatics is as much about computers as cardiology is about stethoscopes. For those who have studied the application of information technologies in medicine, the past decade has delivered one unassailable lesson. Any attempt to use information technology will fail dramatically when the motivation is the application of technology for its own sake rather than the solution of clinical problems.

The role of the information sciences in medicine continues to grow, and the past few years have seen informatics begin to move into the mainstream of clinical practice. The scope of this field is, however, enormous. Informatics finds application in the design of decision support systems for practitioners, in the development of computer tools for research, and in the study of the very essence of medicine—its corpus of knowledge. The study of informatics in the next century will probably be as fundamental to the practice of medicine as the study of anatomy has been this century.

I will consider recent advances in medical informatics with two seemingly contradictory themes in mind—apparently unbridled technological promise against less than satisfying practical achievement—and against three criteria —possibility, practicability, and desirability. Possibility reflects the science of information —what in theory can be achieved? Practicability addresses the potential for successfully engineering a system—what can be built given the constraints of the real world? Desirability looks at the fundamental motivation for using a given technology.

These criteria are suggested because a framework is necessary to judge the claims made for these new technologies by those who seek to profit from them. Just as there is a longstanding symbiosis between pharmaceutical industry and medicine, there is a newer and consequently less examined relation between medicine and the computing and telecommunication industries. Clinicians should try to judge the claims of these newcomers in the same cautious way that they would examine claims about a new drug. Perhaps more so, given that clinicians are far more knowledgeable about pharmacology than they are about informatics and telecommunications.

In this article I will first review recent activities in telemedicine. Since this is a new subject, research themes are only just becoming apparent. Then I will discuss protocol-based decision support systems, which may be the first substantive clinical information system to appear in routine clinical practice. Finally, I will examine the current state of clinical coding. The terminology and coding enterprise is a concerted attempt to describe uniformly the structure, content, and nature of medical knowledge.

Telemedicine

Definitions of telemedicine abound. The essence of telemedicine is the exchange of information at a distance, whether that information is voice, an image, elements of a medical record, or commands to a surgical robot. It seems reasonable to think of telemedicine as the communication of information to facilitate clinical care. And it is not a new enterprise—Einthoven experimented with telephone transmissions using his new invention, the electrocardiograph, at the beginning of the century.

At its inception telemedicine was essentially about providing communication links between medical experts in remote locations. The health care system, however, is clearly inefficient because of its poor communication infrastructure and telemedicine is now seen as a critical way of reducing that cost. One estimate suggests that the health system in the United States could save $30 billion a year with improved telecommunications. Consequently, telemedicine has now become an important subject for research and development. As might be expected, the renewed interest in telemedicine also has much to do with the excitement of new technologies. Currently, the press is flooded with articles about the information superhighway, the Internet, and the rapid growth in the use of mobile telephones. Telemedicine is often presented in the guise of sophisticated new communications technology for specialist activities such as teleradiology and telepathology. These are championed by telecommunication companies because they have the potential to become highly profitable businesses for them. Perhaps influenced by these forces, much of the research in telemedicine is driven by the possibilities of technology rather than the needs of clinicians and patients. Yet the communications infrastructure used by health care will not need to be special. The telecommunications market is competitive and the evolving options are numerous. Health care providers will be able to use the services of cable television, mobile cellular carriers, and telecommunication companies. Furthermore, communications technology does not need to be sophisticated to deliver benefit. Appropriate use of today's telephone can make significant improvements to the delivery of care. For example, follow-up of patients is often possible on the telephone. Rapid communication of hospital discharge information using existing electronic data transfer mechanisms is beneficial for general practitioners. The combined use of mobile telephones and paging systems can reduce the 5-10 minutes out of every hour many clinicians spend answering pagers.

Perhaps more interestingly, inexpensive voice messaging systems can deliver simple but powerful services over existing telephone networks. Voice mail for example, has significant potential for improving the process of care. Leirer et al.

used a voice mail system to phone reminders about drug treatment automatically to elderly people at home, and they showed that it reduced both tardiness and complete forgetting. As more patients get access to electronic mail, this will offer further avenues for innovative health services. Already in some populations, access to electronic mail is high. Fridsma et al. in California found that 46 percent of their patients at clinic already used e-mail, 89 percent of which was through their place of work.

All these points suggest that the potential for the clinical application of communication technologies is indeed great, but equally that there is much still to learn. In particular, the relation between telemedicine and informatics needs to be explored in greater detail. Informatics focuses on the use of information, and telemedicine on its communication. Although seemingly disparate endeavours, they are intimately linked since the goals of communicating information and deciding on its content cannot be separated. Furthermore, there is little clinical value in information systems built simply to gather data for administrators without remembering that the essence of delivering health care is the communication of information between members of the clinical team. Together, the technologies of information and communication can enhance access to information, whether it is stored electronically or is in the possession of a colleague.

Research Issues

Several key research questions are apparent. Firstly, clinical practice already revolves around communication, often by telephone, and important information exchanged in this way is often lost because it is not documented. Capturing the informal information currently lost in health care's communication channels may soon become an important issue for those developing the formal electronic patient record. Deciding what information is important and how that information is made available will require the resolution of issues of confidentiality and security, as well as the technology of storage and retrieval of voice recordings.

Secondly, people's understanding of the effects of technology on communication is still in its infancy. Researchers in human-computer interaction believe that before these technologies can be successfully introduced, the way in which people communicate needs to be understood. In one recent study the presence of a computer during doctor-patient consultations had detectable negative effects on the way doctors communicated. While they were at the computer, doctors gave short responses to patients' questions, delayed responding, glanced at the screen rather than looking at the patient, or structured the interview around the computer rather than the patient. On the positive side, recent experiences in Norway have identified benefits to remote telemedical consultation. Services that provided isolated general practitioners with access to specialist skills had an unexpected side effect. The skills of the general practitioners were increased by repeated interactions with specialists during the management of cases that were previously referred. This may arise through the dynamics of the relationship between a remote general practitioner and a specialist. Unlike in most educational settings, both are motivated to form a coach and apprentice relationship for the immediate management of a patient.

Finally, along with new communication possibilities, come new medicolegal implications. In the United States the courts have decided that radiologists are negligent if they fail to inform clinicians personally of a diagnosis. "Communication of an unusual finding in an x-ray, so that it may be beneficially utilised, is as important as the finding itself." Furthermore, leaving a message with an intermediary is not enough —"certain medical emergencies may require the most direct and immediate response involving personal consultation and exchange." The fact that such communication requirements are beginning to be mandated reflects the community's changing perceptions of best medical practice.

The rapid arrival of telemedicine suggests that the health care community is beginning to identify the benefits of good clinical communications practice and to realise the costs of poor communication. The next few years should see the research in telemedicine mature. The main focus will become the application of communication technologies rather than their development. This represents the same shift in focus that was required of medical informatics, in which initially much effort was spent in developing technologies specifically for medicine.

Protocol-Based Decision Support

Many see the development of protocol-based medicine as the essential cultural change in clinical practice that will permit the design of useful clinical information systems. It was rightly seen as inappropriate for early computer system designers to try to regularise clinical practice to suit the nature of their systems. The move to evidence-based medicine now begins to make it acceptable for clinicians to follow standard assessment and treatment protocols. In this case it is quite appropriate for clinicians to use information systems to help them.

The ultimate goal of a protocol-based decision support system is to provide a set of tools that allows a clinician to access up-to-date guidelines and then apply them to the management of their patients. Simple protocol systems will probably appear in clinical practice by the end of the decade. In some sense, first-generation systems have already appeared as treatment guidelines and clinical trial data can now be accessed on the Internet.

Evidence suggests, however, that even when guidelines are available, clinicians forget to follow them or deviate from them without clear cause. Forgetting preplanned management tasks seems to be especially likely when making clinical decisions in high stress situations. Yet enforcing uniform adherence to guidelines is probably unacceptable, given the complexity of individual cases. It should be possible, however, to make it as easy as possible for clinicians to access guidelines during routine care, making it less likely that steps will be inadvertently forgotten or altered.

This will require the design of more complex systems that will be integrated into the electronic patient record such that protocols can be stored and manipulated by clinicians. For example, best practice recommendations may need to be customised for local conditions or for individual patients. Furthermore, guidelines may be incorporated directly into patient records. As elements of the guideline are completed, they could be automatically noted. The records of care generated in this manner might ultimately be used for population based outcomes analysis...

Terminological Systems

Medical coding systems such as versions of the International Classification of Diseases (ICD), the systematised nomenclature of medicine (SNOMED(30a)), and the Read system(30b) are becoming increasingly familiar to clinicians. Their rationale is as follows. Once captured electronically, clinical data should be available for subsequent aggregation and analysis. However, the words used to describe conditions vary so much that simple analysis is often not possible. Furthermore, the meanings attached to terms may vary. If there was an agreed set of terms to describe the process of care then data analysis would be simplified. The goal of research into medical terminologies is to arrive at a consensus on the most appropriate set of terms and the way they should be structured.

The fundamental advance in terminological research over the past year or so is the realisation that the goal of constructing a complete and universal thesaurus of medical terms is ill posed. Terminology evolves in a context of use, and attempting to define context-independent terminologies is ultimately implausible. Coupled with this view comes the pragmatic understanding that a more robust scientific approach needs to be brought to the enterprise of terminology construction...

The ideal terminological system would be a complete, formal, and universal language that allowed all medical concepts to be described and reasoned about. Some researchers have explicitly asserted that building such a singular and "correct" medical language is their goal. This task emphasises two clear requirements: the ability for the terminological language to cover all the concepts that need to be reasoned about and the independence of the terminology from any particular reasoning task. A further requirement occasionally discussed is that when alternative terminologies exist, they must be logically related such that one can be translated into the other.

Despite the enormous health care investment currently devoted to achieving these goals, current evidence indicates that they are not possible. No set of codes or terms can be universally applied in medicine. There are two fundamental and related obstacles to devising a universal terminological system. The first is the problem that model construction-terminologies are simply a way of modelling the world, and the world is always richer and more complex than any model that humans can devise. The second is the problem of symbol grounding. The words we use to label objects do not necessarily reflect the way we think about the objects, nor do they necessarily reflect defined objects in the real world. The cumulative evidence from recent thinking in cognitive science, computer science, and artificial intelligence provides a formidable set of supporting arguments...

The Way Forward

In the short term, administration agencies keen to obtain aggregate clinical data are driven to adopt existing systems, even if they are imperfect. This has led to much debate among those supporting particular systems of their merits over competing ones.

Doctors in the United Kingdom have been asked to adopt the version 3 Read codes for use not only in personal clinical systems but also in audit, research, outcomes, and guidelines. Such a decision can now be seen to be necessarily interim. What is really needed to help rational choices in the longer term is impartial empirical research, comparing the cost and efficacy of different systems in support of well-defined tasks and contexts. For example, in a recent study comparing the utility of different coding schemes in classifying problem lists from medical records, none of the major systems was found to be comprehensive. The unified medical language system (UMLS) and the systematised nomenclature of medicine were found to be superior to Read and ICD-9 clinical modifications.

In contrast with the British approach, however, the Board of Directors of the American Medical Informatics Association has suggested that it is not necessary or desirable to have all codes coming from a single master system. It suggests that several existing and tested approaches should be embraced, despite their imperfections, in order to progress quickly. A first phase system could be created by borrowing from the different existing code systems, each created for and therefore better suited to different subject domains.

The longer term need will be to introduce more maintainable and extensible systems as the cost of supporting existing systems becomes insupportable. A solution based in part on multiple compositional systems would seem to be most desirable. Since any general medical terminology will cover only a small part of the specific vocabulary of any medical specialty, separate systems may need to be developed for use between and within specialties—"vocabularies need to be constructed in a manner that preserves the context of each discipline and ensures translation between disciplines." Indeed over a century ago, when Farr constructed the classification system ultimately resulting in the ICD, he noted that "several classifications may, therefore, be used with advantage; and the physician, the pathologist, or the jurist, each from his own point of view, may legitimately classify the diseases and the causes of death in the way that he thinks best adapted to facilitate his enquiries."

Specialised compositional systems will thus need to be constructed that agree on a restricted subset of terms necessary for the passage of information between specialties—a kind of Esperanto between different cultures. Work on such communication standards is at present still in its infancy, and more substantive work should be expected in the future. Currently, terms are created without explicit tasks in mind, in the hope that all unseen eventualities will be served. Interspecialty systems would probably need to be tightly task based to ensure maximum utility.

I have reviewed three apparently quite separate areas—

telemedicine, protocol-based decision support systems, and terminologies. They can now be seen to be inextricably entwined since the goals of communicating information and deciding on the content of information cannot be separated. Human communication entails information exchange in a context. What is said depends on the intended message, the method used to convey the message, who is speaking, and who is being spoken to. The development of protocol-based systems and their supporting terminological systems is a perfect example of that symbiosis.

Recent advances in medical informatics leave the following conclusions:

- The application of information and communication technologies in health care should be problem rather than technology driven.
- The use of existing communication technologies such as mobile telephones, voice mail, and e-mail may significantly improve delivery of health care.
- Research is needed to understand human communication processes and needs in health care. Clinical information systems have an important role in the delivery of evidence-based clinical practice.
- The appropriate use of computerised protocols can significantly improve clinical outcome.
- Universal and complete clinical coding schemes are unrealisable, and the continued modification of centralised thesauruses may be technically and financially unsustainable.
- Multiple task-specific terminologies developed in conjunction with clinical protocols may offer the most effective and maintainable long-term strategy.

3

Computer Techniques in Hospital Quality Control

COMPUTER TECHNIQUES IN HOSPITAL QUALITY CONTROL

The establishment of a successful quality control programme requires a systematic approach to the collection and management of large amounts of information. This information must be collected as it is generated because it is too expensive to retrieve it from patient records. The routine analysis of the information may be done on a periodic basis, but there must be a preliminary review to detect events that require immediate intervention. It is this need for timely interventions that make computers invaluable in medical quality control.

Computers are not a substitute for proper administrative procedures, but they are invaluable for performing the repetitive tasks that are intrinsic to an effective quality control programme. For example, the computer can scan each incident report as it is produced to detect specific events, such as an outbreak of a contagious disease. This type of event demands immediate investigation, yet it is very difficult for a quality control manager to take the time to scan every incident report before it is incorporated into the quality control data base. Even in a small facility, where an administrator may be familiar with the entire quality control process, a computer can reduce the chance of overlooking a significant event.

The central management problem in large facilities is the enormity of the data base that must be evaluated. Incident reports must be correlated with infection control data, pharmacy data, and data from many other JCAH mandated oversight committees. The disjointed nature of these reports makes it very difficult to correlate them without the use of computer techniques.

— Types of Techniques
— Data Processing
— Review and Analysis

Types of Techniques

There are three computer techniques that are useful in quality control programmes. The first is data base management or "electronic filing." Data base management includes the creation and updating of computer-based records. These records may be kept solely for quality control purposes, or they may be made accessible for other functions, such as billing. The establishment of an effective data base management system is the first step in establishing a computerized quality control system.

The second technique is the use of statistical tools to analyze quality control data. These tools are necessary to identify legally significant events that may be obscured by the mass of legally insignificant data. There are two types of statistical tools that are useful for analyzing quality control data. The most commonly used tools are descriptive statistics. As the name implies, these tools are used to describe the data, providing information such as averages, means, and so on. The second group of statistical tools involves techniques that measure trends through time.

Trend analysis techniques are important for quality control because they allow the detection of potentially significant events before they result in legal liability. An example of this type of event would be an increasing number of surgical wound infections. While absolute number of infections might still be within allowable limits, a continued increase would push the number of infections into the legally significant area. Such an increase might be obscured by the use of descriptive statistics, but it would be detected by trend analysis.

The third set of techniques involves computer aids to decision making. These techniques range from simple computerized checklists to complex artificial intelligence programmes. The use of computerized checklists is a valuable aid to carrying out preventive law checkups. While checklists are usually too limited for analyzing complex or rapidly changing information, the use of a computer allows the use of branching checklists. These checklists can be made very comprehensive while still remaining easy for unsophisticated personnel to use.

The use of artificial intelligence techniques is still in the experimental stage. A common artificial intelligence technique uses computer programmes that learn from experience. These programmes can survey information for simple patterns, then use the patterns to aid in the detection of more complex patterns. From our experience with these techniques, we believe that their greatest value will be in managing problems such as infection control and medication errors.

Data Processing

The division of quality control activities into simple

tasks is essential to the development of an effective computerized analysis system. The main stumbling block to the effective use of computers in hospitals has been the temptation to computerize all of the hospital's information flow. The have in face been several well-funded attempts to computerize a complete hospital data base (including medical records), but each of these efforts has failed because of the overwhelming amount of data that must be stored and manipulated. In contrast to these attempts. the hospital administrative functions that have been successfully computerized are billing and electronic mail. Both of these functions are simple, requiring no special data handling techniques. They are cost-effective to automate because they are repetitive and provide easily appreciated benefits over manual methods. These are examples of problem-oriented data processing. In each case, the problem to be solved was well-defined and limited in scope.

The use of data processing techniques is crucial to the long-term effectiveness of medical quality assurance programmes. The amount of information that must reviewed to meet current JCAH standards is very large. As these standards tighten, requiring larger amounts of information to be analyzed, it will become impossible to comply with them by manual review techniques. The standards are not onerous, but the growing complexity of health care delivery makes even a cursory analysis of quality control data a massive task.

The problem of managing complex information is not limited to quality assurance activities. Health care providers face this problem in all areas of health care delivery. Just as most hospitals have been forced to automate their billing procedures, they will be forced to automate their quality control efforts, their pharmacy functions, their linen service activities, and all other functions that demand the monitoring of large amounts of data. This automation will be necessary both for economic reasons and to satisfy the hospital's legal duties.

Automated data handling will be legally necessary to document effectively that the hospital is diligent in carrying out its surveillance duties. The hospital is not legally liable for all negligent injuries suffered by patients, only those it could have prevented and those caused by its employees. Thus, to defend itself properly, the hospital must be able to demonstrate that it did in fact monitor the activities of the personnel involved and that this monitoring did not indicate anything untoward that would have alerted the hospital to the necessity for intervention. This monitoring must be more detailed than just reviewing incident reports. It must include a review of all oversight committee function (tissue committee reports, pharmacy committee reports, infection control reports, and so on) to determine if there is a pattern of substandard care. The monitoring must also be sufficiently well-documented to convince a jury that it was conscientiously performed. This demands detailed written records of all surveillance activities.

Review and Analysis

Computer techniques are very useful in the documentation of review functions. The production of proper documentation demands meticulous attention to the detailing of all legally significant events and their disposition. This type of work is difficult to do manually because its repetitive nature leads to errors and low morale. In contrast, the generation of detailed reports is simple in a computer-based system. As an additional benefit, these reports can be archived in a machine-readable form, thereby saving the clerical costs of filing a large volume of written reports.

The basic needs for documentation can be satisfied by computer-generated profiles on the practice of the medical staff, combined with good documentation of the various oversight committee meetings. Most quality control tasks are a matter of assembling and reviewing data with set protocols. It does not make sense to require professional members of an oversight committee to perform this routine data analysis. Such a committee has only a limited amount of time, which is most effectively spent on matters requiring the exercise of professional judgment. It is much more effective to have a computer organise and summarize the necessary data, then have the oversight committee review the processed data.

The lack of appropriate computer resources should not prevent health care providers from using a systems analysis approach to quality control. The most difficult part of automating a task is the identification and simplification of the task. The identification simplification of quality control tasks make it easier to do the task manually and also make the tasks easier to automate in the future. The development of inexpensive, but powerful, small computers has now made it possible for a hospital to utilize several small computers rather than be dependent on one large computer. This simplifies the automation of management functions because the commitment of resources for a microcomputer system is small enough to allow several different systems to be tried. While large computers are still much more powerful than microcomputers, it is often simpler to programme a small dedicated computer than a large system that is devoted to other tasks such as billing. It is also much easier to protect confidential information on a devoted machine than on a remote computer. This is important in preserving medical confidences and in maintaining the legal privilege of investigation reports on legally significant events.

The availability of inexpensive computers, combined with proper management control techniques, allows health care providers in large facilities to manage rationally the mass of quality control information that such facilities generate.

Grid Technology Aids Hospital's Diagnostics

Using grid technology, the hospital's director of the Brain Tumor Research Programme was able to reduce the time it took a text-mining application to run from more than 24 hours to just less than an hour and 20 minutes. Aside from tapping internal resources, Bremer says he expanded his research capabilities and speeded results without adding significant cost, maintenance and IT burdens.

"Our overall goal is to define better diagnostics and therapies for kids with brain tumors. We wanted to lift the human barrier to working with such vast amounts of data within realistic time frames," he says.

Bremer last year rolled out LexiQuest Mine, a data-mining application from SPSS, to start pulling relevant information out of 125,000 document abstracts from 21 medical journals. With more than five years of research at his fingertips, he says he thought LexiQuest Mine would help him more quickly classify brain tumors in patients.

The software lets researchers ask questions, extract concepts and relate the analysis to known brain tumor diagnosis criteria such as gene lists. LexiQuest Mine helped the doctor query and retrieve documents, but more importantly mine the text for concepts. For example, the analytics software understands how groups of words work together such as clinical trial vs. failed clinical trial. Text mining would deliver more accurate results than, say, a search programme.

COMPUTERIZED PHYSICIAN ORDER ENTRY (CPOE) WITH CLINICAL DECISION SUPPORT SYSTEMS (CDSSS)

Medication errors and *adverse drug events* (ADEs) are common, costly, and clinically important problems. Two inpatient studies, one in adults and one in pediatrics, have found that about half of medication errors occur at the stage of drug ordering, although direct observation studies have indicated that many errors also occur at the administration stage. The principal types of medication errors, apart from missing a dose, include incorrect medication dose, frequency, or route. ADEs are injuries that result from the use of a drug. Systems-based analysis of medication errors and ADEs suggest that changes in the medication ordering system, including the introduction of *computerized physician order entry* (CPOE) with *clinical decision support systems* (CDSSs), may reduce medication-related errors.

Despite growing evidence and public mandates, implementation of CPOE has been limited. The Leapfrog Group, a consortium of companies from the Business Roundtable, has endorsed CPOE in hospitals as one of the 3 changes that would most improve patient safety in America. A Medicare Payment Advisory Commission report suggested instituting financial incentives for CPOE implementation. US Senators Bob Graham (D-Fla.) and Olympia Snowe (R-Maine) recently introduced a bill, entitled the "Medication Errors Reduction Act of 2001," to establish an informatics system grant programme for hospitals and skilled nursing facilities. In addition, California recently enacted legislation stipulating that acute care hospitals implement information technology, such as CPOE to reduce medication-related errors.

Practice Description

CPOE refers to a variety of computer-based systems of ordering medications, which share the common features of automating the medication ordering process. Basic CPOE ensures standardized, legible, complete orders by only accepting typed orders in a standard and complete format. Almost all CPOE systems include or interface with CDSSs of varying sophistication. Basic clinical decision support may include suggestions or default values for drug doses, routes, and frequencies. More sophisticated CDSSs can perform drug allergy checks, drug-laboratory value checks, drug-drug interaction checks, in addition to providing reminders about corollary orders (e.g., prompting the user to order glucose checks after ordering insulin) or drug guidelines to the physician at the time of drug ordering.

At times, CDSSs are implemented without CPOE. Isolated CDSSs can provide advice on drug selection, dosages, and duration. More refined CDSSs can incorporate patient-specific information (for example recommending appropriate anticoagulation regimens), or incorporate pathogen-specific information such as suggesting appropriate anti-infective regimens. After viewing such advice, the physician proceeds with a conventional handwritten medication order.

Prevalence and Severity of the Target Safety Problem

It is estimated that over 770,000 people are injured or die in hospitals from ADEs annually. The few hospitals that have studied incidence rates of ADEs have documented rates ranging from 2 to 7 per 100 admissions. A precise national estimate is difficult to calculate due to the variety of criteria and definitions used by researchers. One study of preventable inpatient ADEs in adults demonstrated that 56% occurred at the stage of ordering, 34% at administration,

6% at transcribing, and 4% at dispensing. In this study, the drug class most commonly associated with preventable ADEs was analgesics, followed by sedatives and antibiotics. Even fewer studies have been conducted in the outpatient setting. One recent cross-sectional chart review and patient care survey found an ADE rate of 3% in adult primary care outpatients.

Opportunities for Impact

Clear data do not exist about the prevalence of CPOE with CDSSs or isolated CDSSs. One survey of 668 hospitals indicated that 15% had at least partially implemented CPOE. A slightly more recent survey of pharmacy directors at 1050 acute care hospitals in the United States (51% response rate) reported that 13% of hospitals had an electronic medication order-entry system in place, while an additional 27% stated they were in the process of obtaining such a system.

Study Designs

The first study, a randomized controlled trial evaluating the utility of CPOE in improving prescribing for corollary orders, was conducted by the Regenstrief Institute for Health Care (affiliated with the Indiana University School of Medicine). The remaining 3 studies evaluated the CPOE system at Brigham and Women's Hospital (BWH). Of note, both the Regenstrief and BWH systems are "home-grown" rather than "off-the-shelf" commercial systems. The first BWH study was a cross-sectional analysis comparing an intervention period of CPOE with CDSSs for adult inpatients on medical, surgical, and intensive care wards with a historical period. The other 2 BWH studies were time series analyses of orders written for adult inpatients. Hunt et al updated an earlier systematic review, and included 68 studies that prospectively evaluated use of CDSSs in a clinical setting by a healthcare practitioner with a concurrent control. Importantly, Hunt et al included studies of outpatient settings in their review. Walton's review addressed 15 articles that studied computerized advice on drug dosage for inpatients. Evans et al, at Latter Day Saints Hospital, performed the other 2 studies, again on a "home-grown" system. The first was a randomized controlled trial of empiric antibiotic selection using CDSSs. The second study was a cross-sectional analysis comparing an intervention period of a computer-assisted management programme for anti-infectives with a historical control period. This second study was likely excluded from the systematic review by Hunt et al for methodologic reasons, as it did not have a concurrent control. The reasons for excluding the first study remain unclear. Finally, it is important to emphasize again that of the primary studies that were included, 6 of 8 were performed at 3 institutions with sophisticated "home-grown" systems.

Study Outcomes

Adverse drug events (ADEs), (injuries that result from the use of drugs) by definition constitute clinical outcomes (Level 1). ADEs that are associated with a medication error are considered preventable, while those not associated with a medication error (e.g., known medication side effects) are considered non-preventable. An example of a preventable ADE is the development of rash after the administration of ampicillin to a known penicillin-allergic patient. In contrast, a non-preventable ADE would be development of an ampicillin-associated rash in a patient with no known drug allergies. Non-intercepted serious medication errors include non-intercepted potential ADEs and preventable ADEs (i.e., medication errors that either have the potential or actually cause harm to a patient).

Medication errors refer to errors in the processes of ordering, transcribing, dispensing, administering, or monitoring medications, irrespective of the outcome (i.e., injury to the patient). One example is an order written for amoxicillin without a route of administration. Other medication errors have a greater potential for patient harm and so are often designated as "serious medication errors" or "potential ADEs"—e.g., an order for amoxicillin in a patient with past anaphylaxis to penicillin.

Potential ADEs may or may not be intercepted before reaching the patient. An example of an intercepted potential ADE would be an order written for an acetaminophen overdose that is intercepted and corrected by a nurse before reaching the patient. An example of a non-intercepted potential ADE would be an administered overdose of acetaminophen to a patient who did not suffer any sequelae.

Medication errors include a mixture of serious medication errors with a significant potential for patient injury (Level 2) and other deviations from recommended practice that do not have a clear or established connection to adverse events (Level 3). Examples of the latter include failure to choose the optimal dosing schedule for a medication and many standards related to monitoring serum drug levels and routine electrolytes.

Only 2 studies (from a single institution) evaluating CPOE with CDSSs included ADEs as a secondary outcome (Level 1), and even these studies primary outcomes were serious medication errors (Level 2) and non-intercepted medication errors. The other studies reported a variety of other errors often involving mixtures of Level 2 and Level 3 outcomes—e.g., "prescribing practices" and "corollary orders." *Corollary orders* refer to orders required to detect or ameliorate adverse reactions that may result from the trigger order—e.g., checking the serum creatinine a minimum of 2 times per week in a patient receiving a nephrotoxic agent such as amphotericin. Many corollary orders capture Level 3 outcomes, as failure to prescribe these orders would in most cases have no clear impact on clinical outcomes—e.g., failure to order daily tests for fecal occult blood in patients on heparin or screening audiometry for patients receiving vancomycin.

The predominance of Level 2 and 3 outcomes in these studies is understandable, given the much higher frequency of these outcomes compared to actual ADEs and the enormous costs of conducting these studies.

Similarly, the studies evaluating CDSSs reported a mixture of outcomes from Levels 1-3. Hunt et al reviewed articles to determine changes in patient outcomes (Level 1) or physician performance (Levels 2 and 3, depending on the practice). Walton et al evaluated a range of outcomes (Levels 1-3), including reductions in "adverse reactions and unwanted effects" (Level 1). In one study, Evans et al determined rates of pathogen susceptibility to an antibiotic regimen (Level 2); another study by the same authors evaluated adverse drug events caused by anti-infectives as a main outcome (Level 1).

Evidence for Effectiveness of the Practice

Of the 2 studies at BWH that addressed the impact of CPOE with CDSSs on medication errors and ADEs, the first demonstrated a 55% decrease in serious medication errors. As a secondary outcome, this study found a 17% decrease in preventable ADEs, which was not statistically significant. The second study, a time series analysis, demonstrated marked reductions in all medication errors excluding missed dose errors and in non-intercepted serious medication errors. The number of ADEs in this study was quite small—25 in the baseline period and 18 in the third of the 3 periods with CPOE and CDSS. Correcting for the number of opportunities for errors, the total number of ADEs/1000 patient days decreased from 14.7 to 9.6 ($p=0.09$). For the sub-category of preventable ADEs, the reduction (from 5 to 2) achieved borderline statistical significance ($p=0.05$).

Overhage et al and Teich et al studied more focused aspects of the medication system. Overhage et al studied computerized reminders for corollary orders (e.g., entering a laboratory order to check electrolytes when ordering potassium for a patient) and showed a greater than 100% improvement in the rate of corollary orders ($p<0.0001$). Teich et al studied a broad range of computerized clinical decision support tools utilized at BWH and demonstrated 5 prescribing improvements in types, doses, and frequencies of drug usage.

In summary, these studies provide some evidence that CPOE with CDSSs can substantially decrease medication errors in broad as well as in more focused areas. Despite the significant impact on medication errors, the reduction in ADEs did not achieve statistical significance in one study, and achieved only borderline significance in one of the outcomes in the other study. Furthermore, the systems evaluated in this relatively small literature were developed internally rather than purchased and installed, so the potential impact of commercially available systems remains somewhat speculative.

In the studies evaluating CDSSs, 2 were systematic reviews. In Hunt's review, which emphasized clinical performance, 6 of 14 studies reported improvements in patient outcomes and 43 of 65 studies showed improvement in physician performance. This study concludes that CDSSs can enhance clinical performance for drug dosing, preventive care, and other aspects of medical care, but that the impact of CDSSs on patient outcomes remains unclear. Walton's systematic review evaluated computerized drug dosage advice and found a 6% decrease in adverse drug reactions. The authors concluded that there is some limited evidence that CDSSs for drug dosing are effective, however there are relatively few studies, many of which are of sub-optimal quality. They also suggest that further research is needed to determine if the CDSS benefits realised with specialist applications can be realised by generalist use. Evans et al performed the remaining 2 studies. The 1994 study evaluated the use of a computerized antibiotic selection consultant, and demonstrated a 17% greater pathogen susceptibility to an antibiotic regimen suggested by a computer consultant versus a physician ($p<0.001$). The second study demonstrated a 70% decrease in ADEs caused by anti-infectives ($p=0.018$) through use of a computer based anti-infective management programme. As with CPOE, these CDSSs studies demonstrate improvements in medication errors with statistical significance. In addition, both Walton's systematic review and the latter study by Evans et al demonstrated significant decreases in ADEs. Importantly, each of these CDSSs studies only addressed focal aspects of the medication system. In addition, relatively little information is available about the differences between systems.

Potential for Harm

Faulty decision support data, for example an incorrect default dosing suggestion, can lead to inappropriate ordering choices by physicians. The BWH time series analysis demonstrated an initial rise in intercepted potential ADEs due to the structure of the ordering screen for potassium chloride. This structural error was identified and easily rectified, but underscores the importance of close scrutiny of all aspects of CPOE screens, both initially and on an ongoing basis.

Also, analogously to writing an order in the wrong patient chart in a conventional system, a physician can electronically write an order in the wrong patient's record—e.g., after walking away from the terminal, opening the wrong record from a personalized rounding list. In addition, it is critical that the trigger level for warnings appropriately balances alarm sensitivity and specificity. These systems must have thresholds set so that physicians receive warnings in situations with a potential for significant harm, without being overwhelmed by "false alarms." Another potential risk is hardware outage or software instability. For example, the reliability that is needed with CPOE is much higher than that required for systems that simply report laboratory results.

Costs and Implementation

Six of the studies described in this review evaluated "home-grown" rather than "off-the-shelf" systems. The present costs for purchasing commercial systems are substantially more than the previous costs of developing such systems. For BWH, the cost of developing and implementing CPOE in 1992 was estimated to be $1.9 million, with maintenance costs of $500,000 per year. In comparison, the cost of purchasing and implementing large commercial systems varies substantially, but may be on the order of tens of millions of dollars. Several studies demonstrate that only minimal resources are needed to introduce and/or maintain decision support programmes into existing order entry programmes.

Relatively few data are available regarding the financial benefits of CPOE, although they extend well beyond medication-related events. The net savings of the BWH system are estimated at $5-10 million per year. It is estimated that the costs to BWH for preventable ADEs are $2.8 million annually. Evans et al reported a $100,000 per year cost avoidance with a computer-assisted antibiotic dosing programme largely attributable to decreased antibiotic use and avoided ADEs.

Importantly, healthcare systems must garner both financial and organisational support before introducing CPOE with CDSSs. CPOE requires a very large up-front investment with more remote, albeit substantial returns. In addition, CPOE impacts clinicians and workflow substantially. Its complexity requires close integration with multiple systems, such as the laboratory and pharmacy systems. Failure to attend to the impact of such a large-scale effort on organisational culture and dynamics may result in implementation failure. Therefore, it is essential to have organisational support and integration for its successful implementation and use.

Comment

The literature supports CPOE's beneficial effect in reducing the frequency of a range of medication errors, including serious errors with the potential for harm. Fewer data are available regarding the impact of CPOE on ADEs, with no study showing a significant decrease in actual patient harm. Similarly, isolated CDSSs appear to prevent a range of medication errors, but with few data describing reductions in ADEs or improvements in other clinical outcomes. Finally, the studied CDSSs address focused medication use (for example, antibiotic dosing) rather than more general aspects of medication use.

Further research should be conducted to compare the various types of systems and to compare "home-grown" with commercially available systems. Such comparisons are particularly important since the institutions that have published CPOE outcomes have generally been those with strong institutional commitments to their systems. Whether less committed institutions purchasing "off the shelf" systems will see benefits comparable to those enjoyed by "pioneers" with home-grown systems remains to be determined. Studying the benefits of such complex systems requires rigorous methodology and sufficient size to provide the power to study ADEs. Further research also needs to address optimal ways for institutions to acquire and implement computerized ordering systems.

LABORATORY INFORMATION SYSTEM

A laboratory information system (LIS), is a class of software which handles receiving, processing and storing information generated by Medical laboratory processes. These systems often must interface with instruments and other information systems such as hospital information systems (HIS). An LIS is a highly configurable application which is customized to facilitate a wide variety of laboratory workflow models. Deciding on an LIS vendor is a major undertaking for all labs. Vendor selection, if done properly, should take months of research and planning. Installation takes from a few months to a few years depending on the complexity of the organisation. These are complex software applications which comprise hundreds of tables and critical definitions to build, validate and maintain. There are as many variations of LISs as there types of lab work. Some vendors offer all components, others specialize in specific modules. Disciplines of laboratory science include hematology, chemistry, immunology, blood bank (Donor and Transfusion Management), surgical pathology, anatomical pathology, flow cytometry and microbiology. This article mainly covers clinical lab which encompasses hematology, chemistry and immunology.

Basic Operation

Laboratory Information Systems are often part of an integrated informatics system which involve many disparate applications. Use of an LIS is a critical piece of the clinical IT spectrum of systems and contributes significantly to the overall care given to patients. The LIS is used in inpatient and outpatient settings and in many cases is designed to support both. From an outpatient/ambulatory perspective, LIS interaction frequently begins after a physician has arrived at an initial diagnosis. For example, a patient enters the hospital looking pale and complaining of fatigue. The physician, suspecting anemia, might decide to order a complete blood count (CBC). In an inpatient setting when that patient is admitted into the hospital, the system is called upon often by many in the healthcare industry to order tests, provide specimen processing assistance, receive the results from instrumentation and report on the patient testing in a timely and easy to review manner.

Order Entry and Check In

An order is placed in the system usually by a physician, physician's assistant, nurse, office clerk or laboratory technologist. The order or lab request contains a request of tests to be performed. In many cases, each order is tracked with a unique identifier. This identifier (which is usually a number) is called many things by many systems and is most prominently referred to as an accession. In this hypothetical case, a CBC is ordered which is a panel of sub tests including white blood cell count, red cell blood count and other blood-related tests.

A phlebotomist will be called upon to collect the specimen(s) from the patient. Often, different specimens will be collected, so as to provide a different tubes, with a specific cap color, for each analyser that will process the samples. In this case, the appropriate specimen (Lavender top tube) is taken from the patient, labeled with a bar code specimen label produced by the LIS. The LIS will print barcoded labels (with the unique accession) for the draw tubes. In some cases, more advanced LIS products will also provide a unique identifier for each specimen. This provides the ability to track, at the specimen level, the chain of custody from the point it is taken from the patient to the point that it gets discarded. The specimen-accession-patient hierarchy is linked in a tree like numeric structure. In other cases, the patient is identified by a Patient-ID, and the Sample-ID is linked to the patient's demographic record through the Patient-ID.

Lab Reporting

Lab Reports are the final output of all LIS systems and, in many cases, the primary LIS interaction with healthcare professionals outside of the lab. They can either be printed or faxed in paper-based labs, or delivered via email, file or HL7 interface in paperless installations. The degree to which an LIS supports customizable lab reports and flexibility in modes of delivery of results is one major factor in determining its success in the marketplace.

Specimen Receiving

After the specimen is collected, it is sent/brought to the appropriate lab for processing typically in a batch. This event should be recorded in the LIS. Upon reception in the appropriate testing lab, either manual or automated lab work can begin. CBCs are performed by automated anaylzers.

Results Entry

When results of lab tests are available, they are entered into the system manually or automatically downloaded from an instrument. Once these results are double checked by the medical technologist or autoverified, they are released. Released results are often automatically printed to lab reports which are delivered to the attending physician. LIS systems often provide additional resulting functions and patient care assistance by providing Delta Checking and Reflex Testing functionalities.

Send Test Orders to Analysers

Most LIS systems can be configured to download the specimen data to an analyser either after the order is placed or when a specimen is received in a testing lab. When the barcoded specimen is read by the instrument, the unique ID is read off the specimen label and matched with the order previously downloaded to the instrument. This system is often called "Batch Download". A more efficient system is called "Host Query", where the instrument reads the barcode on the specimen and "queries" the LIS for the test orders. The LIS will be listening on a communication port for queries and will download the requests only when required.

Basic Features

Laboratory Information Systems commonly support the following features:

- Patient Check In
- Order Entry
- Specimen Processing
- Result(s) Entry
- Reporting
- Patient Demographics
- Physician Demographics

Additional Features

In addition LISs commonly support the following:

- Web based order entry
- Web based results inquiry
- Faxing and emailing of lab reports
- Custom report creation
- HL7 interfaces with reference labs and EMRs
- Preliminary reporting
- Final reporting
- Med tech worksheets
- Workload balancing
- Medicare medical necessity checking
- Billing
- Public health reporting
- Rule engines

REDUCING ERRORS IN THE INTERPRETATION OF PLAIN RADIOGRAPHS AND COMPUTED TOMOGRAPHY SCANS

Misinterpretation of radiographic studies is a common source of medical error in both the inpatient and outpatient arenas. Of particular concern is the significant number of misinterpretations of plain radiographs and cranial computed tomography (CT) scans in emergency departments (ED) or urgent care settings by non-radiologists. The prevalence of this patient safety issue may result from the large volume of patients receiving these radiologic tests, which are often done outside normal working hours when radiologists are not available to provide an initial interpretation. This chapter focuses on practices to reduce non-radiologists' higher rates of misinterpretation of these commonly ordered studies.

Intuitively, it would seems that institutions could minimize the number of such mistakes by routinely having studies interpreted by the most accurate and experienced physicians, usually radiologists. The American College of Radiology (ACR) recommends that all imaging procedures culminate in a written, expert opinion from a radiologist or another licensed physician specifically trained in diagnostic radiology. However, due to the associated costs, fewer than 20% of hospitals have full-time on-site coverage by a board-certified radiologist. Instead, radiologists are generally available for 8 to 12 hours a day and may not provide an interpretation until the following morning, particularly when studies are performed after normal working hours. For many routine examinations, it may be possible to delay interpretation without harm to patients. If results are needed urgently and a radiologist is unavailable, other physicians (e.g., emergency physicians, hospitalists, neurologists) must take responsibility for the initial interpretation.

Patient safety may be enhanced by improving the diagnostic accuracy of these physicians or by implementing other systems to prevent initial misinterpretations from adversely affecting patient care. Several strategies reviewed here that may be effective in reducing these errors include educational courses to improve the diagnostic accuracy of non-radiologists, on-site coverage by radiology residents, and mandatory subsequent reinterpretation of studies by radiologists.

Another approach that deserves mention is to have the initial readings made by off-site radiologists or other specialists using a *teleradiology link*. Teleradiology has been effective in facilitating emergent neurosurgical consultation prior to the interhospital transfer of patients with head injury. Teleradiology also allows rural physicians to obtain remote consults for selected patients, which in one report led to treatment changes in 26% of cases. Despite teleradiology's impact in these two specific settings, few studies have tested its accuracy and utility in more general circumstances. Teleradiology of course requires the use of digitized rather than film-based radiographs. In two mixed case series, discrepancies of interpretation between digitized and original radiographs occurred in approximately 10% of cases, with significant discrepancies in 1.5-5%. For more subtle findings the sensitivity of on-screen images may be as low as 49%, leading several investigators to conclude that teleradiology is inferior to film interpretation for difficult cases. At present, it appears that image quality is the major reason behind the variable performance of teleradiology. Although the ACR has established detailed standards for equipment and image resolution, radiology practices often utilize less expensive alternatives for viewing images, including personal computers. The variation in practice, rapid evolution of technology, and lack of large prospective trials make it difficult to examine teleradiology from the standpoint of patient safety. Therefore, this chapter will not discuss teleradiology in detail; reviews can be found elsewhere.

Interventions to improve the technical quality of imaging studies, such as ensuring proper patient positioning and film exposure, are certainly important but are also outside the scope of this chapter. Finally, although radiologists make mistakes in interpreting films, this chapter focuses on practices to reduce the higher rate of misinterpretations made by non-radiologists.

Practice Descriptions

Training Courses

Training courses for non-radiologists are presumably common, but we could locate only 2 descriptions in the literature. Both courses concerned interpretation of cranial CT scans, were conducted by radiologists, and targeted ED residents and faculty physicians. The training lasted 1-2 hours and consisted of a review of neuroanatomy and a small library of CT scans. Two continuous quality improvement initiatives were also recently described, in which radiologists provided regular feedback to ED physicians about their radiograph interpretations.

Initial Interpretations by Radiology Residents

Initial interpretation of ED films by radiology residents follows no standardized practice. Their hours of coverage and the degree to which they interact with ED physicians vary widely. It is also unclear to what extent emergency physicians rely on the resident interpretations when they are available.

Review of All Studies by Radiologists

Reinterpretation of all studies by a radiologist is already commonly used. When a radiologist finds that a study was initially misinterpreted, the medical error has already occurred. In this case, the safety practice concerns how the radiologist communicates the corrected interpretation to providers in order to minimize the risk of harm to patients. The method of communication varies among healthcare facilities and includes placing the interpretation in the patient's medical record, sending a report to the referring physician, or contacting the physician or patient directly for more urgent concerns.

Prevalence and Severity of the Target Safety Problem

Many investigators have focused on the prevalence of all ED readings that are discordant with radiologists' subsequent interpretations (with the radiologists' interpretation assumed to be the "gold standard"). Against this standard, ED physicians and residents misinterpret 1-16% of plain radiographs and approximately 35% of cranial

CT scans. However, many discordant readings involve subtle or incidental findings that are not clinically significant (i.e., they do not affect patient management or outcome). From the standpoint of patient safety, it is the rate of clinically significant misinterpretations and related errors in management that are of concern.

Most ED studies show that important errors in interpretation occur in 1-3% of plain radiographs. However, one pediatric study calculated a 6.8% rate of significant radiograph misinterpretation. The most common error is failure to recognize an extremity fracture. Lufkin and colleagues examined the readings of 16,410 consecutive radiographs and the effect of emergency physicians' confidence on the accuracy of their interpretations. When ED physicians were confident in their interpretation, the rate of discordant readings was 1.2%. More importantly, the rate of clinically significant errors was only 0.1%.

Rates of misinterpretation are even higher for CT scans. In one study, ED residents and attending physicians overlooked new infarcts, mass lesions, and cerebral edema, as well as parenchymal, subarachnoid, and subdural hemorrhages. The rate of clinically important errors was 20-25%, with failure to recognize a cerebral infarction the most common. It is unclear how many patients had adverse outcomes as a result, but the authors estimated that less than 1% of patients were managed inappropriately by ED staff. Other studies confirm that the radiographic accuracy of non-radiologists in detecting a major cerebral infarction is poor, with misinterpretation rates of 30-40%. This may directly impact patient outcomes since management of suspected stroke, specifically determining eligibility for thrombolytic therapy, requires an immediate and accurate interpretation of the CT. In addition, intraobserver and interobserver reliability are fair to poor, with kappa (k) values ranging from 0.41-0.20.

Radiology residents have better accuracy in interpretation of cranial CT scans, though not as high as that of certified radiologists. As part of a departmental quality control programme, Lal and colleagues found the rate of significant misinterpretations by radiology residents was 0.9%. Roszler et al reported moderate or major errors in 2.1% of resident interpretations of post-traumatic head CT scans. Wysoki and colleagues found that major discrepancies between the interpretations of residents and staff radiologists occurred in 1.7% of neuroradiologic studies and that the rate was significantly higher when CT scans were abnormal rather than normal (12.2% vs. 1.5%). Residents missed 9% of intracranial hemorrhages and 17% of cranial or facial fractures.

Opportunities for Impact

The accepted standard of care, supported by the ACR, calls for routine review of all radiologic studies by a radiologist or other qualified physician in a timely fashion. Given the available data on staffing patterns, we estimate that on-site radiologists are available to interpret radiographs about half the time. Radiologists generally read any remaining studies the following day. In academic centers, the percentage of films initially interpreted by residents may range from 20% to 100%, and the availability of on-call residents is highly variable. It is also unclear what proportion of academic and community hospitals provides radiographic training courses for non-radiologists.

Study Designs

Few studies specifically focus on methods to reduce clinically significant misinterpretations of radiographs and

CT scans. No randomized trials have evaluated the effectiveness of the 3 patient safety practices identified above.

Study Outcomes

Most studies reported the rate of clinically significant misinterpretations (Level 2 outcome). However, the definition of "clinically significant" was subjective and varied among reports. One trial reported only the percentage of correct CT interpretations (Level 3), without describing the significance of specific errors.

Evidence for Effectiveness of the Practices

Levitt and colleagues found a significant improvement in cranial CT scan interpretations by ED physicians after a one-hour training course. However, there were several limitations of this study. The intervention was not tested before implementation, raising concerns regarding its reliability and reproducibility. Previously published research at the same institution showed a 38.7% misinterpretation rate of cranial CT scans by ED physicians. Because physicians were aware of these results, they may have engaged in their own efforts that led to improvement in CT scan interpretation. The improvement might also be explained by significant changes in case-mix, which was not measured. A multicenter study by Perron et al showed that a reproducible educational course significantly improved residents' ability to interpret CT scans. However, the study is limited by possible selection bias (participation in the course was voluntary; post-test data were obtained in only 61 of 83 subjects). Although subjects in the study by Perron were retested after a 3-month washout period, neither course has been shown to result in sustained improvement. Quality improvement programmes such as those described by Espinosa and Preston successfully reduced the rate of misinterpreted radiographs and number of callbacks, respectively. Through ongoing feedback and review of misinterpreted radiographs, Espinosa and colleagues lowered the rate of important errors from 3% to 0.3%, a relative risk reduction of 90%. The initiative described by Preston led to a 42.9% relative reduction in callbacks to the ED, although the absolute magnitude was less impressive (0.3% absolute risk reduction).

We found no studies that compared the readings of ED physicians with those of radiology residents in a real-world environment. Only one investigation compared their diagnostic skill in an experimental situation. Eng and colleagues exposed 4 groups of physicians (ED attendings, ED residents, radiology attendings, and radiology residents) to a series of 120 radiographs and calculated their receiver operating characteristic (ROC) curves. The radiographs were selected for their difficulty, and ED physicians had previously misinterpreted many of them. The area under the ROC curve was 0.15 higher for radiology faculty than for ED attendings (95% CI: 0.10-0.20) and 0.07 higher for all faculty than all residents (95% CI: 0.02-0.12). Compared with ED faculty, radiology residents had an additional area under the ROC curve of 0.08 (95% CI: 0.02-0.14).

Potential for Harm

There is a potential for both radiologists and non-radiologists to overread films (i.e., falsely identify non-existent findings), which may result in unnecessary diagnostic testing or treatment. Since the vast majority of this literature considers the radiologist's reading to be the gold standard, the proportion of discrepancies in interpretation that are due to false-positive readings by radiologists is unclear.

Costs and Implementation

Only one study reported the costs of false-positive

readings by ED physicians, which averaged $85 per false-positive radiograph. Given the paucity of research, it is not possible to estimate the costs of implementing universal review of emergency films by an on-site radiologist. Finally, no studies have measured the costs of misreads to the patient and healthcare system (e.g., transportation, return visits, repeat or unnecessary studies, unnecessary medications) which could potentially offset staffing costs. The marginal costs of after-hours staffing alone may be prohibitive, especially for low-volume sites. No information is available to estimate the cost of establishing a high-quality teleradiology programme, or of educational programmes for ED physicians or trainees.

Comment

The rates of misinterpreted radiographs and CT scans are high in many studies. Of particular concern is the 20-25% rate of clinically significant errors in reading cranial CT scans, even among experienced emergency physicians and neurologists. Although plain films are correctly interpreted more than 90% of the time, even "low" error rates of 1% or less are important given the sheer number of films.

The relative roles of ED physicians, radiology residents, certified radiologists, and other physicians will depend on their accuracy and their cost. The literature is notable for the relative dearth of studies of interventions to reduce radiologic misinterpretation by non-radiologists, even though dozens of studies have documented the problem. Where radiographs must be interpreted by non-radiologists, there is limited evidence that brief educational interventions and continuous quality improvement programmes improve diagnostic accuracy. It is possible that radiologists' routine review of plain radiographs may not be cost-effective when the non-radiologist clinician has a high level of confidence in the initial interpretation, but this has not been rigorously established. Coverage by radiology residents may add back-up accuracy to the reading of an ED attending, but Eng's study was biased toward a difficult set of radiographs that had previously been misinterpreted by emergency physicians. The added value of a radiology resident's interpretation may be much lower in actual practice.

One avenue of research that could yield effective safety practices is human resource management. Essentially, staffing could be optimized such that specific tests could be triaged to the individual with the highest diagnostic accuracy. This kind of intervention would require assessment of both potential coverage gaps and the skill mix of the available labor force. A formal protocol might be developed and tested to identify coverage vulnerabilities and develop realistic coverage options based on measured performance of the available personnel at a particular site. While the value of this strategy is entirely speculative, it draws on general management science and could be explored more explicitly in healthcare.

INFORMATION TRANSFER

Patient safety can be compromised by discontinuities in care. Studies suggest that discontinuity results from poor information transfer and faulty communication, which in turn may cause avoidable adverse events.

Improving information transfer and communications among healthcare providers is an important patient safety practice and has been strongly recommended as a means to improve patient care. This chapter evaluates safety practices involving improvements of provider-to-provider information transfer. Practices for evaluation include transfer of information between inpatient and outpatient pharmacies, sign-out systems for medical housestaff, automatically generated electronic discharge summaries, and systems to improve patient notification of abnormal results.

Information Transfer Between Inpatient and Outpatient Pharmacies

Accurate and timely information transfer between community and acute care pharmacies is an important safety practice. Patients admitted to the hospital could benefit from the hospital's pharmacy obtaining better information concerning their medication allergies as well as prior therapeutic failures. Furthermore, when patients transition from acute care to outpatient care, changes in medications that occurred during hospitalisation may cause confusion for both patients and providers. In one study surveying patients one week after hospital discharge, patients' knowledge of their drug indications were worse for medications introduced during their hospitalisation than for those taken prior to hospitalisation (OR 0.69, 95% CI: 0.53-0.89).

Confusion and incomplete information may increase the risk of under- or overmedication, harmful drug interactions, and other problems. Existing literature suggests that pharmacist interventions may reduce potential adverse drug events and have a modest impact on patient morbidity and mortality. However, these studies have used independent reviewers to judge the impact of the intervention and have not specifically measured adverse drug events or patient outcomes. Clinical pharmacists' consultations prior to discharge might also improve patient medication compliance.

Uncontrolled studies report that information-exchange programmes between hospital and community pharmacies are perceived as beneficial and may have a positive impact on patient outcomes. Although not the primary outcome measured in their small (n=127) observational study, Dvorak et al did note that using a pharmacy-to-pharmacy referral form was effective in preventing 2 medication errors. Thus, practices that improve information transfer between hospital and community pharmacies may improve patient safety.

Of the many potential methods for improving information transfer between hospitals and outpatient pharmacies, controlled trials have been reported in the literature for only 2: pharmaceutical care plans cards and patient information facsimiles between pharmacies. Although direct electronic communication of pharmacy data may be superior to these methods, no controlled studies are currently available regarding this practice and therefore it is not reviewed within this chapter.

Practice Description

In a study by Smith and colleagues, patients received a card prior to discharge listing their pharmaceutical care plan, which included medication doses, indications, schedules, side effects, information as to the importance of drug compliance, and how to obtain medication refills. Patients were instructed to give the card to their community pharmacist. In another study, the intervention consisted of pharmacy-to-pharmacy facsimile transmission at the time of admission and discharge from the hospital. In this study, when a patient was admitted to the hospital their community pharmacy transmitted patient demographic information, historical information concerning allergies and adverse drug reactions, current medications, refill history, pharmacist's monitoring notes, communications with patient and physician, and a detailed medication history to the admitting hospital. After discharge the hospital pharmacy transmitted to the community pharmacy a list of any potential medication problems identified by the hospital pharmacist on admission, the patient's daily monitoring log, the pharmacist's discharge summary, and a discharge medication table. The medical records department of the hospital also transmitted the patient's discharge summary and laboratory test results to the community pharmacy.

Prevalence and Severity of the Target Safety Problem

Medication problems can arise because patients are frequently discharged from the acute care hospital on medications different from their ambulatory regimen. Elderly patients in particular are at risk after discharge. In one study, hospital providers changed 53% of the drugs prescribed by the primary care providers.

The extent to which these medication changes and lack of communication result in recently discharged patients failing to receive medications or appropriate monitoring for their drug therapy is unclear. In one study of elderly patients, 32% of medications prescribed at discharge were not being taken 2 days after discharge. Another study found that 51% of patients recently discharged from acute care hospitals had deviated from their prescribed regimen. Of those that had deviated from the prescribed drug regimen, 70% did not understand the medication regimen. In a Scottish study, recently discharged, elderly patients were issued a 5-day supply of their medication on discharge and visited in their homes after these 5 days had elapsed. Twenty-seven percent of the patients had not received a new prescription ordered on discharge. Of the patients with new prescriptions issued, 19% received inaccurately labeled medications. Medications were considered mis-labeled when non-specific container labels, such as "take as directed" replaced the more specific labels given on discharge. Some authors have suggested that improving communication about medications prior to and just after hospital discharge might reduce these medication errors.

Poor communication is not the only problem. Patient factors influence whether a medication is ultimately picked up and taken as directed. Deviations from prescribed drug regimens are multifactorial and improving pharmacy-to-pharmacy communication is only one aspect of the overall problem.

Opportunities for Impact

Data from primary care providers reveal that 96% of the respondents would like information concerning hospital drug changes. Ninety-four percent of community pharmacists surveyed also wished to be provided with information concerning hospital drug changes. We were unable to identify data regarding what percentage of hospital pharmacies routinely transfer information on patients' medication regimens when they are admitted to and discharged from acute care.

Study Design and Outcomes

Two controlled studies were identified in the literature. Both were randomized trials but neither was blinded. In Smith et al, patients received a written pharmacy care plan at discharge. Home visits were made 7 to 10 days later to assess compliance and discrepancies in the medication that patients were taking versus those ordered at discharge (Level 2). In the study by Kuehl et al, patients were randomly assigned to either usual care or to a bi-directional exchange of pharmacy information by facsimile between the ambulatory pharmacy and the admitting hospital, upon admission and discharge (Level 1). The outcomes were pharmacist interventions, such as changing medication doses or making allergy recommendations.

Evidence for Effectiveness of the Practice

Smith et al's small study (n=53) of a pharmacy care plan card found that in both groups patients were taking different medications than those ordered at discharge. The authors found that compliance with post-discharge medications was significantly better in the group that had received the information card ($p<0.01$). Unintentional changes to the medication were found in 14/28 (50%) of the study patients and 17/25 (68%) of the control patients during the follow-up visits (Pearson's chi-square $p=0.18$)

In the study by Kuehl et al, significantly more experimental group patients than control group patients had at least one in-hospital pharmacist intervention documented (47% vs. 14%, $p<0.001$). The mean number of in-hospital pharmacist interventions per patient was also significantly higher in the experimental group (1.0 vs. 0.2, $p<0.0001$). The types of interventions made by hospital pharmacists included addition of a medication the patient was taking as an outpatient that was not originally ordered on admission, dosage changes, and changes related to drug allergy. Interventions by ambulatory care pharmacists were also more frequent in experimental group patients compared with control group patients. Community pharmacists who received hospital pharmacy records performed interventions on one or more patients 42% of the time, while no interventions were performed in the control group ($p=0.001$). Specific community pharmacist interventions included monitoring of therapy (13/57), taking actions related to drug allergy problems (13/57), requesting documentation of an indication for a particular medication (9/57), and making a dosage change (8/57).

Although the data abstractor was blinded with regard to study group, the nature of the intervention did not permit blinding of participating pharmacists (i.e., they received faxed information for some patients but not others). Also, the pharmacists were not explicitly blinded to the study's objectives. It is unclear how this knowledge might have affected the results. It could have resulted in more careful scrutiny of any potential drug problem (bias away from the null) or less scrutiny of these orders (bias towards the null). Kuehl et al note that although the results suggest discriminatory documentation did not play a major role, the possibility cannot be ruled out.

Another potential limitation of this study was the completeness of follow-up. Of the eligible patients from ambulatory care pharmacies, only 50% returned to their pharmacy during the study period. There were no comparisons presented between the ambulatory pharmacy visit group and the loss to follow-up group. This large loss to follow-up could have significantly altered their findings.

Potential for Harm

None of the studies evaluating different hospital-community pharmacy communication processes detailed any adverse events. However, the degree of added workload and effects on current workflow must be taken into account.

Costs and Implementation

The 2 reviewed interventions for improving hospital to community pharmacy information transfer seemed simple and relatively inexpensive. Although no formal cost analysis was performed, Dvorak et al described their method (use of a pharmacy-to-pharmacy referral form) as being "labor-intensive." No records were kept of the time necessary to provide the referrals but the authors estimated the time commitment per patient to be 30 minutes. It is also important to note that complete information transfers occurred for 75% of the subjects in Kuehl's study, indicating that there is still room for improving the process. With improvements in information transfer technology, automated transfer of information from hospital to community pharmacy could have important patient safety benefits without excessively increasing providers' workloads.

Comment

Providing patients with data forms to convey transfer of information between hospital and ambulatory pharmacies has potential for reducing discontinuities resulting from inadequate medication information. Few studies have evaluated the effect of these interventions on patient outcomes, although any improvement in the transfer of this information would likely be well received by ambulatory providers. Future studies are necessary to determine if and how improved pharmacy-to-pharmacy communications reduce preventable adverse drug events and improve patient outcomes. Identifying the most effective and least disruptive forms of inter-pharmacy communication remains an area for further investigation.

COMPUTER ADVERSE DRUG EVENT (ADE) DETECTION AND ALERTS

Adverse drug events (ADEs) occur in both inpatient and outpatient settings. Most institutions use spontaneous incident reporting to detect adverse events in general, and ADEs in particular. Spontaneous incident reporting relies exclusively on voluntary reports from nurses, pharmacists and physicians focused on direct patient care. However, spontaneous reporting is ineffective, identifying only one in 20 ADEs. Efforts to increase the frequency of spontaneous reporting have had only a minor impact.

Several studies demonstrate the effectiveness of using computerized detection and alert systems (referred to as *computer "monitors"*) to detect ADEs. In 1991, Classen et al published information about a computerized ADE monitor that was programmed to identify signals—in effect mismatches of clinical information—that suggested the presence of an ADE. The signals included sudden medication stop orders, antidote ordering, and certain abnormal laboratory values. The computerized signals were then evaluated by a pharmacist who determined whether an ADE had occurred. Based on the rules of this study, Jha et al developed a similar monitor that identified approximately half the ADEs identified by chart review, at much lower cost. Similarly, Bowman and Carlstedt used the Regenstrief Medical Record System to create a computerized inpatient ADE detection system. Compared to the "gold standard" of chart review, the monitor had 66% sensitivity and 61% specificity, with a positive predictive value of 0.34. Finally, one community hospital implemented an ADE monitor with triggers that were reviewed by pharmacists who then contacted physicians to make appropriate regimen changes. This study identified opportunities to prevent patient injury at a rate of 64/1000 admissions. These studies and others demonstrate the potential value of computer monitors, especially when linked to effective integrated information systems. While monitors are not yet widely used, they offer an efficient approach for monitoring the frequency of ADEs on an ongoing basis, and the Health Care Financing Administration is considering mandating them.

Practice Description

Computerized ADE alert monitors use rule sets to search signals that suggest the presence of adverse drug events. The most frequently studied rule sets (or "triggers") are those that search for *drug names* (e.g., naloxone, kayexalate), *drug-lab interactions* (e.g., heparin and elevated PTT) or *lab levels alone* (e.g., elevated digoxin levels) that frequently reflect an ADE. Simple versions can be implemented with pharmacy and laboratory data alone, although the yield and positive predictive value of signals is higher when the 2 databases are linked.

Further refinements include searches for International Classification of Diseases (ICD-9) codes, and text-searching of electronic nursing bedside charting notes or outpatient notes for *drug-symptom combinations* (e.g., medication list includes an angiotensin converting enzyme inhibitor and the patient notes mention "cough"). Although these refinements do increase the yield of monitors, they require linkage to administrative databases or electronic medical records.

The information captured with computer monitors is used to alert a responsible clinician or pharmacist, who can then change therapy based on the issue in question. Systems are designed to alert the monitoring clinician in various ways. Alerts can go to one central location (e.g., hospital pharmacist) or to individual physicians. Monitoring pharmacists typically review the alert and contact the appropriate physician if they determine that the alert has identified a true event. The alert modality also varies based on the available technology, from printed out reports, to automatic paging of covering physicians, to display of alerts on computer systems (either in results or ordering applications). It should be emphasized that computerized physician order entry is not a requirement for these monitors. Thus, a simple version of this approach could be implemented in most US hospitals.

Prevalence and Severity of the Target Safety Problem

It is estimated that over 770,000 people are injured or die in hospitals from ADEs annually, but variations in study criteria and definitions prevent precise national estimates. Fewer data address the epidemiology of ADEs in the outpatient setting. One recent study found an ADE rate of 3% in adult primary care outpatients, while an older study reported a similar rate of 5% among ambulatory patients attending an internal medicine clinic over a 1-year period.

Detection and alerting interventions primarily target ADEs related to the medication ordering process. One study of preventable inpatient ADEs in adults demonstrated that 56% occurred at the stage of ordering. Among the 6.5 ADEs per 100 admissions in this study, 28% were judged preventable, principally by changing the systems by which drugs are ordered and administered. In one study of computerized ADE detection, the ADEs identified by computerized monitoring were significantly more likely to be classified as severe than those identified by chart review (51% vs. 42%, p=0.04). Thus, monitors may capture a subset of events with the most potential for patient injury.

Injuries due to drugs have important economic consequences. Inpatients that suffer ADEs have increased lengths of stay of nearly 2 days and added hospital costs of more than $2000. Bootman has estimated the annual cost of drug-related morbidity and mortality within the United States at $76.6 billion, with the majority ($47 billion) related to hospital admissions due to drug therapy or the absence of appropriate drug therapy.

Opportunities for Impact

Unfortunately, there are no good data as to how many hospitals have integrated lab and medication systems, which are required for many of the triggers used in computerized ADE monitors.

Study Designs

We found 5 studies of computerized ADE alert systems

that were Level 3 or better. Four studies detected potential ADEs using computerized monitoring and then alerted physicians or pharmacists about the event. One additional study both alerted the monitoring clinician and made recommendations for actions relating to the suspect condition. Four studies were in the inpatient setting and one was in the ambulatory setting.

Study Outcomes

All of the studies reported Level 1 or 2 outcomes. Level 1 outcomes were the rate of ADEs and renal impairment (as reflected by rises in creatinine). Level 2 outcomes included percent of time recommended actions were taken and time to respond to an event.

Evidence for Effectiveness of the Practice

One study demonstrated significant decreases in adverse clinical outcomes with the alert systems. This decrease included a surprisingly large reduction in allergic reactions (ones not previously known); it is not clear how the computer alert or decision support system could have contributed to this result. The second study showed no significant difference in the number of adverse events in the intervention and control groups. This study and 3 others revealed significant improvements in response times concerning lab values, and one study found a significant decrease in the risk of serious renal impairment. Finally, one study demonstrated significant changes in physician behaviour/modification of therapy based on alerts with recommended actions.

Potential for Harm

None of the studies discuss any potential for harm associated with the monitor and alerts. It is certainly possible that alerts could be erroneous, but it is doubtful that this would lead to any direct patient harm. As in studies of safety in other industries, one possible source of harm could be too many false positives. Large numbers of clinically insignificant warnings for patients would interfere with routine care, and might result in providers ignoring all warnings, even clinically meaningful ones.

Costs and Implementation

In general, implementation of alert monitors requires computer systems that can link laboratory and medication information. Integrating this information requires the creation of interface between the drug and laboratory databases, with costs that will vary depending on the nature of the existing information systems. In addition, alert methods vary, with some applications directly contracting physicians (which requires further integration of coverage and pager databases) and others using pharmacist intermediaries. The cost of pharmacist review of triggers was less than 1 FTE per hospital in 2 studies; one of them reported an annual cost savings of up to 3 million dollars by reducing preventable ADEs with this alerting technique.

Studies thus far suggest that physicians view computerized alert systems favourably. Forty-four percent of physician-respondents receiving alerts indicated that the alerts were helpful and 65% wished to continue receiving them (although these alerts went to many physicians because it was unclear who the responsible doctor was). In another study in which alerts were sent only to the responsible physician, 95% of physician-respondents were pleased to receive them.

The systems in these studies were all "homegrown" and contained idiosyncrasies that might undermine their implementation elsewhere. Clearly it is important that systems track which physicians are responsible for which patients. In addition, all 4 of the inpatient studies were conducted at tertiary care hospitals and the outpatient study was done at clinics affiliated with a tertiary care center. The translation of this alerting approach to community settings may be difficult. One community teaching hospital has reported success in detecting opportunities to prevent injury (64/1000 admissions) using computerized detection and alerting.

Comment

Computerized real-time monitoring facilitates detection of actual and potential ADEs and notification of clinicians. This in turn may aid in the prevention of ADEs or decrease the chances that ADEs will cause harm. The monitors also yield improvements in secondary measures relating to the length of time until response and the quality of response. The applications in these studies were all "homegrown." Future applications should be evaluated and refined further. In particular, it is important to quantify the yield of collecting these data in terms of patient outcomes, since the start-up costs are significant. If monitors do lead to important clinical benefits, they should become standard features of commercially available hospital computer systems. As this occurs, careful attention will need to be paid to optimizing the response process. In addition, little has been done to translate these monitoring systems to the outpatient setting, largely because outpatient clinical information is often not computerized or resides in disparate systems. As integrated computerized outpatient records become more common, the systems developed in the inpatient setting should be translatable to the outpatient setting.

SIMULATOR-BASED TRAINING AND PATIENT SAFETY

For a number of years, simulators have been used in aviation, nuclear power, military flight operations and other industries as a training tool and method to assess performance. Their use is nearly universal in high reliability organisations. Recently the use of simulation in medicine has increased markedly, in part due to greater awareness of the importance of patient safety.

Defined broadly, a simulator replicates a task environment with sufficient realism to serve a desired purpose. In medical training, simulators can substitute for actual patients and can be as simple as utilizing pigs' feet to practice suturing, or as complex as virtual reality machines and re-creations of actual clinical environments for surgeons, radiologists and anesthesiologists. In a general sense, they improve patient safety by allowing physicians to become better trained without putting patients at risk. For example, in a randomized controlled trial, Peugnet and colleagues used a virtual reality simulator to train physicians to perform retinal photocoagulation and found that surgeons who trained with the simulator performed the procedure as well as those who trained with patients. Gaba lists several other advantages of simulation, among them:

- Presentation of uncommon but critical scenarios in which a rapid response is needed (e.g., malignant hyperthermia, which occurs once in every 40,000 anesthesia cases). To conduct systematic training about managing such critical events there is little alternative but to use simulation.
- Errors can be allowed to occur and reach their conclusion—in real life a more capable clinician would have to intervene—so participants can see the results of their decisions and actions.
- With mannequin-based simulators clinicians can use actual medical equipment, exposing limitations in the human-machine interface.
- Complete interpersonal interactions with other clinical staff can be explored and training in

> teamwork, leadership, and communication provided. In a number of medical fields, simulation has been used in crew resource management (CRM) training, where the focus is on behavioural skills such as inter-team communication during critical incidents.

Human error is a leading cause of adverse anesthesia events that lead to poor patient outcomes and may play an important role in surgical errors as well. However, it may be difficult to demonstrate improved patient outcomes from simulation because adverse events are unusual and there are an extreme number of potential confounders. Given these difficulties, performance has been used as a surrogate outcome, despite concerns that it may be a less than perfect measure. It is yet unclear which attributes of performance matter most to patient outcomes. Additionally, the methods (e.g., reliability and consistency) and timing (e.g., duration of follow-up) by which performance is measured also remain ill-defined. Studies of the effectiveness of simulators often are limited in that they measure performance using the same training simulator, which may favour those who have trained on the simulator itself. In other words, seemingly improved performance may not translate to actual patient care. Of the studies that have extended laboratory simulation to patient care, few have evaluated the impact on medical error or established a clear link between simulator training and patient outcomes.

This chapter reviews the evidence regarding the use of simulators in the training and ongoing education of healthcare providers as a patient safety measure. Not included in this review is the use of simulators in the planning or preparation of diagnostic or therapeutic interventions in specific patients (e.g., calculation of radiotherapy doses using computer simulations, planning a surgical procedure for a specific patient using 3-D simulations based on the anatomical data from the actual patient). While these kinds of simulation clearly decrease the morbidity and mortality associated with their particular procedures, they are omitted here because they focus on unique characteristics of individual patients that may not be generalizable to other patients. Other uses of simulators beyond the scope of this discussion include simulators to measure worker proficiency, to identify areas for educational intervention, and to target improvements in training.

Simulators in Anesthesia

Patient simulators have been most widely studied in anesthesia where human error may account for over 80% of critical incidents. Simulators range from simple mannequins to high-fidelity simulators that recreate the operating room experience. According to one study, 71% of medical schools in Canada, the United Kingdom and other western nations used mannequins or some other form of simulator to teach anesthesia to medical students. There is a growing body of literature on the different roles that simulators can play in anesthesia training.

Studies have found that simulators can effectively identify errors and appropriateness of decision making in anesthesia. For example, during 19 comprehensive anesthesia simulations, DeAnda et al documented 132 unplanned incidents, of which 87 (66%) were due to human error and 32 (27%) were considered critical incidents. Schwid and O'Donnell have also used simulators to document the type of errors that anesthesiologists make in critical incidents, finding errors in monitor usage (37%), airway management (17%), ventilator management (13%), and drug administration (10%). Gaba and colleagues studied both the appropriateness of decisions and response time of anesthesia trainees to simulated critical incidents. They found great individual variability as well as variability by incident in the accuracy and timeliness of response. Some simulated incidents, such as cardiac arrest, had major errors in management a majority of the time. Based on these studies, patient simulators can be used to identify areas for further education or training of anesthesia providers.

We identified 2 studies of the effect of simulators on anesthetists' performance. Schwid and colleagues studied the impact of a computer screen-based anesthesia simulator in a randomized, controlled trial of 31 first-year anesthesia residents. Residents that had trained on the simulator with individualized debriefing responded better to critical events on a mannequin-based simulator than those who received standard training without the simulator. Using a randomized, controlled design, Chopra and colleagues studied management of simulated critical situations by 28 resident or staff anesthesiologists. The performance of subjects who trained on the simulator was superior to that of subjects who did not receive that training.

Another setting where simulators may play an important role is in crew resource management (CRM). Though establishing the effectiveness of simulation in CRM training may be difficult, initial work has been done on reliably and consistently rating performance. Proficiency on a simulator does not ensure proficiency in clinical settings. Simulator fidelity (i.e., how accurately the simulator replicates reality) is imperfect. It is much more difficult to "re-create" a human being than to do so for, say, an airplane. This limitation is illustrated by a study conducted by Sayre and colleagues. They studied emergency medical technicians (EMT) who learned intubation techniques on anesthesia mannequins. After successfully intubating the mannequins 10 times, they were permitted to intubate patients in the field, where their proficiency was only 53%. Other factors can inhibit optimum learning using simulation or the applicability of learning to real practice. Some participants may be more vigilant than usual during simulator sessions. Others may be unable to "suspend disbelief," may treat the simulation only as a game, or act in a cavalier fashion, knowing that the simulator is not a real patient. Refinement of simulators to make them more sophisticated and life-like may help to improve the quality of the training that simulators can provide. Appropriate construction of curricula and debriefings can also minimize the potential problems of simulation training.

Simulators in Radiology

The number of radiologic examinations that require sedation, analgesia, or contrast media has increased rapidly in recent years. Despite their rarity, serious medication reactions do occur and require prompt, appropriate management. Some evidence of suboptimal management has prompted the creation of computer-based simulators to improve training in these areas. Simulators have also been used to measure the effectiveness of strategies to teach trainees about critical incidents, but studies have not reported the effectiveness of simulators as adjuncts to training. Sica and colleagues developed a computer-based simulator that was used to study the effectiveness of a lecture and videotape-based intervention on critical incidents for radiology housestaff. Those residents who underwent the intervention scored better on the simulator than those that had only received basic, standard training. The authors concluded that the simulator was an effective way of assessing the utility of the educational course.

Simulators in Surgery

As surgical technique and expertise has changed drastically over recent decades, some methods used to train surgeons have evolved as well. Simulators in the surgical setting are aimed at improving surgeons' technical skills and dexterity. Training on simulators and virtual reality machines, though still in its nascent stages, is becoming increasingly accepted. Surgical simulators have been developed for a variety of procedures: endovascular repair of abdominal aortic aneurysms, sinus surgery gynecologic surgery, orthopedic surgery, prostatic surgery, amniocentesis procedures, and oral surgery. Nonetheless, many of these have yet to be formally evaluated in terms of efficacy in improving physician performance in patient care.

We identified several studies that evaluated physician performance after training on a surgical simulator. Derossis evaluated surgical residents and attendings in a randomized study and found that those trained with a simulator had greater proficiency in suturing, transferring, and mesh placement, when tested on the simulator, than did the control group. They subsequently found that when tested *in vivo* in pigs, surgeons (both attendings and residents) who had been randomized to the simulator arm were more proficient at the same skills. Scott and colleagues studied the impact of a video-trainer on laparoscopic cholecystectomy skills. They randomized surgical residents to training on a video-trainer versus no formal training over a 30-day period. At the end of the period, when tested on pre-specified tasks on the video trainer, those who trained on the video trainer did uniformly better.

Intuitively, improved technical skills should lead to fewer complications during surgery. Wallwiener and colleagues developed a surgical trainer that, when used in conjunction with other improvements in their training programme, led to lower rates of hysteroscopic complications. However, for most simulators the link between improvements in technical skills and dexterity from simulator training and prevention of adverse events has yet to be established and deserves formal investigation. Further, problem-based surgical simulation (e.g., avoiding inadvertent ligation of the ureter during hysterectomy) may improve patient safety not only by improving skills, but also by training surgeons to better anticipate and avoid complications and to manage them should they occur.

Simulators in Gastroenterology

Simulators have been developed to train physicians in the technical skills required in endoscopy. We identified one study that evaluated the effect of simulator training on physician performance. In a small randomized controlled trial enrolling 10 residents, Tuggy and colleagues found residents who trained for flexible sigmoidoscopy using a virtual reality simulator were faster, visualized a greater portion of the colon, and made fewer directional errors in actual patients.

Simulators in Cardiology

Cardiology training has long used a variety of simulators from audiocassettes of heart tones to full patient simulators. Two simulators have been evaluated. Champagne and colleagues demonstrated that a heart sound simulator could increase medical students' recognition of pathologic heart sounds. Ewy and colleagues studied the efficacy of "Harvey," a cardiology patient simulator. In a study enrolling 208 senior medical students at 5 medical schools, participants were randomized to receive training on Harvey versus a standard cardiology curriculum during their cardiology elective. Students who had been trained with Harvey performed skills better both when tested with the simulator and when tested with real patients. Some physicians have expressed concern that training on simulators may decrease professionalism. In this study, there was no difference in the way patients perceived the professionalism of the students trained on Harvey compared with students who received standard training.

Systems that simulate the cardiovascular anatomy and physiology have also been developed. Swanson and colleagues created a cardiovascular simulator to train physicians on the workings of mechanical valves and balloon assist devices, and to recognized diseased vessels. As cardiac procedures have become more invasive, simulators to train cardiologist in these procedures have become more common, but their effect on resident performance has not been evaluated formally.

Comment

Although simulators have been used for many years in a variety of settings, data on their efficacy are still emerging. While there is currently no evidence that simulation-based training leads to improved patient outcome, it may prove difficult to conduct such studies. These would require large cohorts of patients to be followed during and after care by clinicians who were randomized to have undergone different cumulative amounts of simulation training. Because adverse events are uncommon, and there are a large number of patient-based and system-based factors that contribute to negative outcomes, any such study would have to be massive and prolonged. Instead, provider performance, with its known limitations, has been and will continue to be used as a surrogate outcome. Nonetheless, as Gaba has asserted "...no industry in which human lives depend on skilled performance has waited for unequivocal proof of the benefits of simulation before embracing it." Certain benefits are clear. In training for procedures, simulators have high face validity because they ease trainees' transition to actual patients, which seems inherently beneficial as a means to avoid adverse events.

Further, procedural success is related to the experience of the operator, known as the volume-outcome relationship. As simulators become more advanced, they may be reasonable substitutes to improve proficiency of both trainees and low volume physician operators. This increase in proficiency may have an important impact in patient outcomes. Future studies of the link between simulator-based training and performance on actual patients will improve our ability to better assess the appropriate role of simulators in training and patient safety.

The costs of simulators vary widely and need to be considered. "Home-made" or simple trainers are far less expensive than complex simulators or full-scale simulation centers. The average cost of high-fidelity patient simulators is on the order of $200,000. Medium fidelity simulators may be as little as $25,000. Establishing a dedicated simulation center can cost up to $1,000,000 (including the simulator) depending on the amount of space, the type of clinical equipment to be used, the extent of renovations needed, and the sophistication of the audio-visual equipment. However, such capital costs are amortized over a long period of time, and such centers typically are used for a wide variety of training curricula for diverse target populations. Further, for most simulation training the dominant cost is that of instructor time. Another indirect cost is that of removing clinical personnel from revenue producing work to undergo training. The healthcare industry currently does not fully embed time or costs of training into the system, but instead often leaves these costs for the individual clinicians to bear. There are potential risks to simulation-based training. Where the simulator cannot properly replicate the tasks or task environment of caring for patients, there is a risk that clinicians might acquire inappropriate behaviours (negative training) or develop a false sense of security in their skills that could theoretically lead to harm. Although there are no data to suggest that this currently happens, such risks will have to be weighed and evaluated as simulators become more commonly used.

In summary, although there is currently little evidence that simulation training improves patient care, the experience with simulation in other industries and the high face validity of their applications in healthcare has led many institutions to adopt the technology. It is likely that simulators will continue to be used and their role in training of medical personnel will grow. Definitive experiments to improve our understanding of their effects on training will allow them to be used more intelligently to improve provider performance, reduce errors and ultimately, promote patient safety. Although such experiments will be difficult and costly, they may be justified to determine how this technology can best be applied.

4

Hospital and Health Communication System

HOSPITAL AND HEALTH COMMUNICATION SYSTEM

Hospital Communication System

Hill-Rom Company, a subsidiary of Hillenbrand Industries, Inc., is the world's leading manufacturer of patient care products. Hill-Rom's COMposer Communication System is a comprehensive communication and information management system designed to enhance the quality of care that hospitals provide to their patients. The system offers direct room-to-room communication, instant location of staff members, and activity reports showing patient call records and response times. When a patient calls for a nurse, the master station provides the responding staff member with background information about the patient, thereby ensuring a personalized response to every call.

The wall-mounted stations enable staff members to locate each other and communicate directly between any two stations in the network. Both types of station are equipped with a control wheel that gives the workstations a simple, non-intimidating appearance. Rotating the control wheel sequentially highlights all available options on the associated computer display, thereby eliminating guesswork and errors. Corridor lights allow staff to identify quickly which patient in a semi-private room is calling, which rooms have nurses in them, and which rooms have some type of emergency in progress. Staff members wear transmitter badges that enable the system to locate them and direct calls to the nearest communication station.

American Institutes for Research worked closely with Hill-Rom to ensure the usability of COMposer. We joined the project at an early stage of needs definition and concept development. From that point on, we worked with Hill-Rom's project team to (1) develop a conceptual model suited to the needs of first-time users as well as people using the system for several years, (2) establish the mechanics of interaction, and (3) design a comprehensive set of software screens. At several stages of the project, we prototyped the user interface of system components and evaluated them by means of usability test.

Picture archiving and communication system

In medical imaging, picture archiving and communication systems (PACS) are computers or networks dedicated to the storage, retrieval, distribution and presentation of images.

Types of PACS

Full PACS handle images from various modalities, such as ultrasonography, magnetic resonance imaging, positron emission tomography, computed tomography, endoscopy, mammography and radiography (plain X-rays).

Small-scale systems that handle images from a single modality (usually connected to a single acquisition device) are sometimes called *mini-PACS*.

Uses

PACS replaces hard-copy based means of managing medical images, such as film archives. It expands on the possibilities of such conventional systems by providing capabilities of off-site viewing and reporting (distance education, tele-diagnosis). Additionally, it enables practitioners at various physical locations to peruse the same information simultaneously, (teleradiology). With the decreasing price of digital storage, PACS systems provide a growing cost and space advantage over film archives. PACS is offered by virtually all the major medical imaging equipment manufacturers. There are also several PACS open-source projects. The most difficult area for PACS systems is interpreting the DICOM image format which is slightly variably implemented between different radiology equipment vendors. The ability to point the tags in the DICOM format coming from vendors equipment to useable titles in a PACS is a feature common to most vendors and software offerings.

Architecture

Typically a PACS network consists of a central server which stores a database containing the images. This server is connected to one or more clients via a LAN or a WAN which provide or utilize the images. Web-based PACS is becoming more and more common: these systems utilize the Internet as their means of communication, usually via VPN or SSL. The software (thin or smart-client) is loaded via ActiveX, Java, or .NET Framework. Definitions vary, but most claim that for a system to be truly web based, each individual image should have its own URL. Client workstations can use local peripherals for scanning image films into the system, printing image films from the system and interactive display of digital images. PACS workstations offer means of manipulating the images (crop, rotate, zoom, brightness, contrast and others).

Modern radiology equipment, modalities, feed patient images directly to the PACS in digital form. For backwards compatibility, most hospital imaging departments and radiology practices employ a film digitizer. The medical images are stored in an independent format. The most common format for image storage is DICOM (Digital Imaging and Communications in Medicine), a NEMA standard.

Integration

A full PACS system should provide a single point of access for images and their associated data (i.e. it should support multiple modalities). It should also interface with existing hospital information systems: hospital information system (HIS) and radiology information system (RIS).

Interfacing between multiple systems provides a more consistent and more reliable dataset:

— Less risk of entering an incorrect patient ID for a study – modalities that support DICOM worklists can retrieve identifying patient information (patient name, patient number, accession number) for upcoming cases and present that to the technologist, preventing data entry errors during acquisition. Once the acquisition is complete, the PACS can compare the embedded image data with a list of scheduled studies from RIS, and can flag a warning if the image data does not match a scheduled study.

— Data saved in the PACS can be tagged with unique patient identifiers (such as a social security number or NHS number) obtained from HIS. Providing a robust method of merging datasets from multiple hospitals, even where the different centers use different ID systems internally.

An interface can also improve workflow patterns:

— When a study has been reported by a radiologist

the PACS can mark it as read. This avoids needless double-reading. The report can be attached to the images and be viewable via a single interface.

— Improved use of online storage and nearline storage in the image archive. The PACS can obtain lists of appointments and admissions in advance, allowing images to be pre-fetched from nearline storage (for example, tape libraries or DVD jukeboxes) onto online disk storage (RAID array).

Recognition of the importance of integration has led a number of suppliers to develop fully integrated RIS/PACS systems. These may offer a number of advanced features:

— Dictation of reports can be integrated into a single system. The recording is automatically sent to a transcriptionist's workstation for typing, but it can also be made available for access by physicians, avoiding typing delays for urgent results, or retained in case of typing error.

— Provides a single tool for quality control and audit purposes. Rejected images can be tagged, allowing later analysis (as may be required under radiation protection legislation). Workloads and turn-around time can be reported automatically for management purposes.

History

The principles of PACS were first discussed at meetings of radiologists in 1982. Various people are credited with the coinage of the term *PACS*. Cardiovascular radiologist Dr Andre Duerinckx reported in 1983 that he had first used the term in 1981. Dr Samuel Dwyer, though, credits Dr Judith M. Prewitt for introducing the term.

COMMUNICATING

Every clinical action, every treatment choice and investigation, is shaped by the available information. We can think of this information as the clinical evidence that is used to make a judgement about the right course of action. Clinicians gather evidence through communication with others, either through what is said now, or what has been documented from before.

There are many different sources of clinical evidence that can be used in the routine care of a patient, and these include:

- The patient, who will give information about their symptoms and their problems, as well as demonstrate clinical signs through physical examination,
- The clinical literature, which captures past knowledge about disease and treatment,
- The patient record, which records the history of a patient's state, both based upon clinical observation and laboratory and imaging reports, as well as their various treatments and the impact of treatment on their disease,
- Clinical measurement devices, from the simple like a blood pressure cuff, through to the complex such as a glucometer, cardiogram or multi-probe patient monitor in intensive care,
- Clinical colleagues, who may exchange messages containing information about the state of patients, their opinions, their own workload and needs, or clinical knowledge.

The information contained in these clinical "messages" comes in a variety of media and formats and can be delivered in a variety of ways including face-to-face conversations, letters, e-mail, voicemail, and electronic or paper medical records.

When this exchange of information works well, clinical care is solidly based upon the best evidence. When information exchanges are poor, the quality of clinical care can suffer enormously. For example, the single commonest cause of adverse clinical events is medication error, which account for about 19% of all adverse events, and the commonest prescription errors can be redressed by the provision of better information about medications or the patients receiving them (Bates et al, 2001). Poor presentation of clinical data can also lead to poorly informed clinical practice, inappropriate repeat investigation, unnecessary referrals, and wastes clinical time and other resources (Wyatt and Wright, 1998). In this chapter we will look at the communication process and explore how variations in the structure of clinical messages affect the way in which they are interpreted, and therefore affect the quality of care. If the motto for Chapter One was "A map is not the territory" then the motto for this Chapter is "the chart is not the patient".

The Structure of M message Determines how it will be Understood

What a message is meant to say when it is created, and what the receiver of a message understands, may not be the same. This is because what humans understand is profoundly shaped by the way data are presented to us, and by the way we react to different data presentations. Thus it is probably as important to structure data in a way so that it can be best understood, as it is to ensure that the data are correct in the first place. What a clinician actually understands after seeing the data in a patient record and what the data actually shows are very different things. For example, the way data are structured has a profound effect on the conclusions a clinician will draw from the data. The data show preliminary results from two hypothetical clinical trials of a generic "conventional treatment" compared with a generic "investigational treatment", both treating the same condition. In an experiment to see if clinicians would decide to stop the trial because the data show one of the treatments was obviously better than the other, the decision to stop varied significantly depending upon how the data were displayed. Correct decisions were significantly more common with icon displays (82%) and tables (68%) than with pie charts or bar graphs, both 56%.

If this example was reflected in actual clinical practice, up to 25% of the patients treated according to data displayed as bar or pie charts would have received inappropriate treatment. Consequently, there is an enormous difference between simply communicating a message to a colleague, and communicating it effectively.

The message that is sent may not be the message that is received

Messages are misunderstood both because of the limitations of the agents interpreting them, and because the very process of communication itself is limited. To explore the nature of communication, we will develop a general model that describes the process of sending a message between two agents. The agents might be two human beings, or a human and a computer. A communication act occurs between the two agents A1 and A2 when agent A1 constructs a message m1 for some specific purpose, and sends m1 to agent A2 across a *communication channel*.

The second agent A2 receives a message m2, which may in some ways be different from the intended message m1. The effectiveness of the communication between the agents is dependent upon several things—the nature of the channel, the state of the individual agents, the knowledge possessed by the agents, and the context within which the agents find themselves.

Communication Channels Distort Messages

A wide variety of different communication channels are available to us, from the basic face-to-face conversation, through to telecommunication channels like the telephone or e-mail, and non-interactive channels like the medical record.

The message is sent as a signal down the channel, and the message signal may be corrupted because of limitations in the channel bearing the message. For example, faxed or photocopied documents may be harder to read than digitally transmitted documents because of poor resolution and distortion of the transmitted document.

Channels vary in their *capacity* to carry data, and the more limited the channel capacity, the less of the original message can be transmitted at any one time. Simply put, the thinner the channel 'pipe', the less data can flow through at any given moment.

The signal to noise ratio *measures how much a particular message has been corrupted by noise that has been added to it during transmission across a channel.*

Channels also have different abilities to send a message exactly as it was sent, and often the message is distorted in transmission. This distortion is usually called *noise*. Noise can be thought of technically as any unwanted signal that is added to a transmitted message while being carried along a channel, and distorts the message for the receiver. So, noise can be anything from the static on a radio, to another conversation next to your own, making it hard to hear your partner—one person's signal is another's noise. Standard information theory describes how the outcome of a communication is determined in part by the capacity and noise characteristics of a channel.

So, we note that in general, when an agent sends a message, the message may be modified by the channel, and be received as a slightly different message by the receiving agent.

Individuals don't know the same things

In Chapter two we saw that the inferences that can be drawn from data are dependent on the knowledge used to make the inference. Since different individuals 'know' slightly different things, they will usually draw different inferences from the same data because of this variation in their individual knowledge. Thus variations in diagnosis and treatment decisions, based upon the same data, may simply reflect the differences in clinical knowledge between individual clinicians.

However, when sending a message, we have to make assumptions about the knowledge that the receiver has, and use that to shape our message. There is no point in explaining what is already known, but it is equally as important to not miss out important details that the receiver should know to draw the right conclusions. Thus notionally identical messages sent to a clinical colleague or to a patient end up being very different because we assume that the colleague has more common knowledge, and requires less explanation, than the patient. The knowledge shared between individuals is sometimes called *common ground* (Coiera, 2000).

This explains why individuals communicate more easily with others that have similar experiences, beliefs and knowledge. Intuitively we know that it takes greater effort to explain something in a conversation to someone with whom we share less common background. Conversely, individuals who are particularly close can communicate complicated ideas in terse shorthand. One of the reasons agents create common ground is to optimise their interaction. By sharing ground, less needs to be said in any given message, making the interaction less costly.

With this in mind, we can now say that each agent possesses knowledge about the world, in the form of a set of models *K*. Critically, the private world models of the two communicating agents in our model, K1 and K2, are not identical. Thus agent A1 creates a message m1, based upon its knowledge of the world K1. A2 receives a slightly different message m2 because of channel effects, and then generates its own private interpretation of the message's meaning based upon its own knowledge K2. Further, agent A1 makes a guess about the content of K2, and shapes its message to include data or knowledge it believes agent A2will need to make sense of the message being sent. The effectiveness of the message is dependent upon the quality of the guess an agent can make about what the receiving agent knows. Usually, agents send more than is needed, because some redundancy in a message improves the chance that what the receiver needs is actually sent.

HEALTH COMMUNICATION

Use Communication Strategically to Improve Health.

Health communication encompasses the study and use of communication strategies to inform and influence individual and community decisions that enhance health. It links the domains of communication and health and is increasingly recognized as a necessary element of efforts to improve personal and public health. Health communication can contribute to all aspects of disease prevention and health promotion and is relevant in a number of contexts, including (1) health professional-patient relations, (2) individuals' exposure to, search for, and use of health information, (3) individuals' adherence to clinical recommendations and regimens, (4) the construction of public health messages and campaigns, (5) the dissemination of individual and population health risk information, that is, risk communication, (6) images of health in the mass media and the culture at large, (7) the education of consumers about how to gain access to the public health and health care systems, and (8) the development of telehealth applications.

For individuals, effective health communication can help raise awareness of health risks and solutions, provide the motivation and skills needed to reduce these risks, help them find support from other people in similar situations, and affect or reinforce attitudes. Health communication also can increase demand for appropriate health services and decrease demand for inappropriate health services. It can make available information to assist in making complex choices, such as selecting health plans, care providers, and treatments. For the community, health communication can be used to influence the public agenda, advocate for policies and programmes, promote positive changes in the socioeconomic and physical environments, improve the delivery of public health and health care services, and encourage social norms that benefit health and quality of life.

The practice of health communication has contributed to health promotion and disease prevention in several areas. One is the improvement of interpersonal and group interactions in clinical situations (for example, provider-patient, provider-provider, and among members of a health care team) through the training of health professionals and patients in effective communication skills. Collaborative relationships are enhanced when all parties are capable of good communication.

Another area is the dissemination of health messages through public education campaigns that seek to change the social climate to encourage healthy behaviours, create awareness, change attitudes, and motivate individuals to adopt recommended behaviours. Campaigns traditionally have relied on mass communication (such as public service announcements on billboards, radio, and television) and educational messages in printed materials (such as pamphlets) to deliver health messages. Other campaigns have integrated mass media with community-based programmes. Many campaigns have used social marketing techniques.

Increasingly, health improvement activities are taking advantage of digital technologies, such as CD-ROM and the World Wide Web (Web), that can target audiences, tailor messages, and engage people in interactive, ongoing exchanges about health. An emerging area is health communication to support community-centered prevention Community-centered prevention shifts attention from the individual to group-level change and emphasizes the empowerment of individuals and communities to effect change on multiple levels.

A set of Leading Health Indicators, which focus on key health improvement activities and are described in *Healthy People 2010: Understanding and Improving Health*, all depend to some extent on effective health communication. The promotion of regular physical activity, healthy weight, good nutrition, and responsible sexual behaviour will require a range of information, education, and advocacy efforts, as will the reduction of tobacco use, substance abuse, injuries, and violence. For example, advocacy efforts to change prices and availability of tobacco and alcohol products have resulted in lower consumption levels. Effective counseling and patient education for behaviour change require health care providers and patients to have good communication skills.

Public information campaigns are used to promote increased fruit and vegetable consumption (5-A-Day for Better Health!), higher rates of preventive screening (mammogram and colonoscopy), higher rates of clinical preventive services (immunization), and greater rates of adoption of risk-reducing behaviours.

Health communication alone, however, cannot change systemic problems related to health, such as poverty, environmental degradation, or lack of access to health care, but comprehensive health communication programmes should include a systematic exploration of all the factors that contribute to health and the strategies that could be used to influence these factors. Well-designed health communication activities help individuals better understand their own and their communities' needs so that they can take appropriate actions to maximize health.

Issues and Trends

The environment for communicating about health has changed significantly. These changes include dramatic increases in the number of communication channels and the number of health issues vying for public attention as well as consumer demands for more and better quality health information, and the increased sophistication of marketing and sales techniques, such as direct-to-consumer advertising of prescription drugs and sales of medical devices and medications over the Internet. The expansion of communication channels and health issues on the public agenda increases competition for people's time and attention;

at the same time, people have more opportunities to select information based on their personal interests and preferences. The trend toward commercialization of the Internet suggests that the marketing model of other mass media will be applied to emerging media, which has important consequences for the ability of noncommercial and public health-oriented health communications to stand out in a cluttered health information environment.

Communication occurs in a variety of contexts (for example, school, home, and work); through a variety of channels (for example, interpersonal, small group, organisational, community, and mass media) with a variety of messages; and for a variety of reasons. In such an environment, people do not pay attention to all communications they receive but selectively attend to and purposefully seek out information. One of the main challenges in the design of effective health communication programmes is to identify the optimal contexts, channels, content, and reasons that will motivate people to pay attention to and use health information.

A one-dimensional approach to health promotion, such as reliance on mass media campaigns or other single-component communication activities, has been shown to be insufficient to achieve programme goals. Successful health promotion efforts increasingly rely on multidimensional interventions to reach diverse audiences about complex health concerns, and communication is integrated from the beginning with other components, such as community-based programmes, policy changes, and improvements in services and the health delivery system. Research shows that health communication best supports health promotion when multiple communication channels are used to reach specific audience segments with information that is appropriate and relevant to them. An important factor in the design of multidimensional programmes is to allot sufficient time for planning, implementation, and evaluation and sufficient money to support the many elements of the programme. Public-private partnerships and collaborations can leverage resources to strengthen the impact of multidimensional efforts. Collaboration can have the added benefit of reducing message clutter and targeting health concerns that cannot be fully addressed by public resources or market incentives alone.

Research indicates that effective health promotion and communication initiatives adopt an audience-centered perspective, which means that promotion and communication activities reflect audiences' preferred formats, channels, and contexts. These considerations are particularly relevant for racial and ethnic populations, who may have different languages and sources of information. In these cases, public education campaigns must be conceptualized and developed by individuals with specific knowledge of the cultural characteristics, media habits, and language preferences of intended audiences. Direct translation of health information or health promotion materials should be avoided. Credible channels of communication need to be identified for each major group. Television and radio serving specific racial and ethnic populations can be effective means to deliver health messages when care is taken to account for the language, culture, and socioeconomic situations of intended audiences.

An audience-centered perspective also reflects the realities of people's everyday lives and their current practices, attitudes and beliefs, and lifestyles. Some specific audience characteristics that are relevant include gender, age, education and income levels, ethnicity, sexual orientation, cultural beliefs and values, primary language(s), and physical and mental functioning. Additional considerations include their experience with the health care system, attitudes toward different types of health problems, and willingness to use certain types of health services. Particular attention should be paid to the needs of underserved audience members.

Targeting specific segments of a population and tailoring messages for individual use are two methods to make health promotion activities relevant to audiences. Examples include the targeted use of mass media messages for adolescent girls at increased risk of smoking; the tailoring of computer-generated nutritional information to help individuals reduce their fat intake and increase fruit and vegetable consumption; and a national telephone service for Spanish speakers to obtain AIDS information as well as counseling and referrals.

Interventions that account for the cultural practices and needs of specific populations have shown some success. For example, a breastfeeding promotion programme among Navajo women that was based on investigations of their cultural beliefs about infant feeding practices showed increased rates of breastfeeding. Similarly, an intervention that used the novela, a popular form of Latino mass media, to reach young people and their parents sought to improve parent-youth communication in Hispanic families and to influence the adolescents' attitudes about alcohol.

Advances in medical and consumer health informatics are changing the delivery of health information and services and are likely to have a growing impact on individual and community health. The convergence of media (computers, telephones, television, radio, video, print, and audio) and the emergence of the Internet create a nearly ubiquitous networked communication infrastructure. This infrastructure facilitates access to an increasing array of health information and health-related support services and extends the reach of health communication efforts. Delivery channels such as the Internet expand the choices available for health professionals to reach patients and consumers and for patients and consumers to interact with health professionals and with each other (for example, in online support groups).

Compared to traditional mass media, interactive media may have several advantages for health communication efforts. These advantages include (1) improved access to personalized health information, (2) access to health information, support, and services on demand, (3) enhanced ability to distribute materials widely and update content or functions rapidly, (4) just-in-time expert decision support, and (5) more choices for consumers. The health impact of interactivity, customization, and enhanced multimedia is just beginning to be explored, and already interactive health communication technologies are being used to exchange information, facilitate informed decisionmaking, promote healthy behaviours, enhance peer and emotional support, promote self-care, manage demand for health services, and support clinical care.

Widespread availability and use of interactive health communication and telehealth applications create at least two serious challenges. One is related to the risks associated with consumers' use of poor quality health information to make decisions. Concerns are growing about the Web making available large amounts of information that may be misleading, inaccurate, or inappropriate, which may put consumers at unnecessary risk. Although many health professionals agree that the Internet is a boon for consumers because they have easier access to much more information than before, professionals also are concerned that the poor quality of a lot of information on the Web will undermine informed decisionmaking. These concerns are driving the development of a quality standards agenda to help health professionals and consumers find reliable Web sites and health information on the Internet. An expert panel convened by the U.S. Department of Health and Human Services describes high quality health information as accurate, current, valid, appropriate, intelligible, and free of bias.

The other challenge is related to the protection of privacy and confidentiality of personal health information. The personal privacy and the confidentiality of health information are major issues for consumers, and these concerns are magnified when information is collected, stored, and made available online. As the availability and variety of interactive health applications grow, consumer confidence about developers' ability or intent to ensure privacy will be challenged. In the near future, personal health information will be collected during both clinical and nonclinical encounters in disparate settings, such as schools, mobile clinics, public places, and homes, and will be made available for administrative, financial, clinical, and research purposes. Although public health and health services research may require de-identified personal health information, policies and procedures to protect privacy will need to ensure a balance between confidentiality and appropriate access to personal health information.

The trend of rapidly expanding opportunities in health communication intersects with recent demands for more rigorous evaluation of all aspects of the health care and public health delivery systems and for evidence-based practices. Numerous studies of provider-patient communication support the connection among the quality of the provider-patient interaction, patient behaviour, and health outcomes. As the knowledge base about provider-patient interactions increases, a need becomes apparent for the development of practice guidelines to promote better provider-patient communication. Additional evidence about the process of health information-seeking and the role of health information in decisionmaking also is needed. Health communication campaigns could benefit as well from more rigorous formative research and evaluation of outcomes. Expected outcomes should be an important consideration and central element of campaign design. As health communication increasingly involves electronic media, new evaluation approaches are emerging. Given the critical role that communication plays in all aspects of public health and health care, health communication and outcomes research should become more tightly linked across all health communication domains.

Because national data systems will not be available in the first half of the decade for tracking progress, one subject of interest concerning health communication is not addressed in this focus area's objectives. Representing a research and data collection agenda for the coming decade, the topic covers persons who report being satisfied with the health information they received during their most recent search for such information. Health-conscious consumers increasingly are proactive in seeking out health information. Individuals want information about prevention and wellness as much as about medical problems. Public health and the medical community share an interest in promoting—and sustaining—informed decisions for better health. Surveys suggest that people want to get health information from a professional and that counseling by health professionals can be effective both in reducing lifestyle risks and supporting self-management of chronic diseases like diabetes. However, diminished time in clinical visits and some clinicians' discomfort with open communication work against optimum information exchange. In addition, many people want information to be available when and where they need it most. Health information should be not only easily accessible but also of good quality and relevant for the needs of the person. The increasing use of the Internet as a source for health information will require greater awareness of the importance of the quality of information.

Disparities

Often people with the greatest health burdens have the least access to information, communication technologies, health care, and supporting social services. Even the most carefully designed health communication programmes will have limited impact if underserved communities lack access to crucial health professionals, services, and communication channels that are part of a health improvement project.

Research indicates that even after targeted health communication interventions, low-education and low-income groups remain less knowledgeable and less likely to change behaviour than higher education and income groups, which creates a knowledge gap and leaves some people chronically uninformed. With communication technologies, the disparity in access to electronic information resources is commonly referred to as the "digital divide." The digital divide becomes more critical as the amount and variety of health resources available over the Internet increase and as people need more sophisticated skills to use electronic resources.] Equitably distributed health communication resources and skills, and a robust communication infrastructure can contribute to the closing of the digital divide and the overarching goal of Healthy People 2010 to eliminate health disparities.

Even with access to information and services, however, disparities may still exist because many people lack health literacy. Health literacy is increasingly vital to help people navigate a complex health system and better manage their own health. Differences in the ability to read and understand materials related to personal health as well as navigate the health system appear to contribute to health disparities. People with low health literacy are more likely to report poor health, have an incomplete understanding of their health problems and treatment, and be at greater risk of hospitalization. The average annual health care costs of persons with very low literacy (reading at the grade two level or below) may be four times greater than for the general population. An estimated 75 percent of persons in the United States with chronic physical or mental health problems are in the limited literacy category. People withchronic conditions, such as asthma, hypertension, and diabetes, and low reading skills have been found to have less knowledge of their conditions than people with higher reading skills. Although the majority of people with marginal or low literacy are white native-born Americans, changing demographics suggest that low literacy is an increasing problem among certain racial and ethnic groups, non-English-speaking populations, and persons over age 65 years. One study of Medicare enrollees found that 34 percent of English speakers and 54 percent of Spanish speakers had inadequate or marginal health literacy.As the U.S. population ages, low health literacy among elderly people is potentially a large problem. Nearly half of the people in the elderly population have low reading skills, and reading ability appears to decline with age. A study of patients 60 years and older at a public hospital found that 81 percent could not read and understand basic materials such as prescription labels and appointments.

Opportunities

For health communication to contribute to the improvement of personal and community health during the first decade of the 21st century, stakeholders, including health professionals, researchers, public officials, and the lay public, must collaborate on a range of activities. These activities include (1) initiatives to build a robust health information system that provides equitable access, (2) development of high-quality, audience-appropriate information and support services for specific health problems and health-related decisions for all segments of the population, especially underserved persons, (3) training of health professionals in the science of communication and the use of communication technologies, (4) evaluation of interventions, and (5) promotion of a critical understanding and practice of effective health communication.

A national health information infrastructure (NHII) provides a framework that stakeholders can use to communicate with each other and to transform data into useful information on multiple levels. Efforts are under way throughout the world to develop integrated national and global health information infrastructures to support health improvements. In the United States, the National Committee on Vital and Health Statistics (NCVHS) is advising the Secretary of Health and Human Services and Congress on the health information needs of the country. The NCVHS defines NHII as all of the technologies, standards, applications, systems, values, and laws that support individual health, health care, and public health. Issues related to technical standards, privacy and confidentiality, and regulatory guidelines are being addressed by the public and private sectors.

The infrastructure makes it possible for people not only to use health information designed by others but also to create resources to manage their own health and to influence the health of their communities. For example, community groups could use computers to gain access to survey information about the quality of life in their neighborhoods and apply this information to create an action plan to present to local elected and public health officials. Information is a critical element of informed participation and decisionmaking, and appropriate, quality information and support services for all are empowering and democratic.

As patients and consumers become more knowledgeable about health information, services, and technologies, health professionals will need to meet the challenge of becoming better communicators and users of information technologies. Health professionals need a high level of interpersonal skills to interact with diverse populations and patients who may have different cultural, linguistic, educational, and socioeconomic backgrounds. Health professionals also need more direct training in and experience with all forms of computer and telecommunication technologies. In addition to searching for information, patients and consumers want to use technology to discuss health concerns, and health professionals need to be ready to respond. To support an increase in health communication activities, research and evaluation of all forms of health communication will be necessary to build the scientific base of the field and the practice of evidence-based health communication.

Many health care organisations and public service agencies use the Internet as one of their main channels for information delivery. Access to the Internet and subsequent technologies is likely to become essential to gain access to health information, contact health care organisations and health professionals, receive services at a distance, and participate in efforts to improve local and national health. The integration of communication media means electronic access to health information not only via computers but also with Web-enabled televisions and telephones, handheld devices, and other emerging technologies. Technical literacy, or the ability to use electronic technologies and applications, will be essential to gain access to this information.

Internet availability in the home is an important indicator of equitable access among population groups. An increasing number of people have access to the Internet at work and public facilities, such as libraries and community centers, but several limitations affect the use of online health information and support in these settings. Some employers monitor electronic mail and the types of sites visited by employees. Access in public settings may be problematic because of privacy and confidentiality concerns, and access may be needed during times when these facilities are unavailable. Because of the potentially sensitive nature of health-related uses of the Internet, access at home is essential.

Although the proportion of people with access to the Internet has risen dramatically since 1995, many segments of the population lack access, such as low-income and rural households; persons with less education; and certain racial and ethnic groups, such as African Americans and Hispanics. Internet access rates vary considerably according to income. Only 11 percent of households earning $24,999 or less have access, whereas 19 percent are connected among those earning $25,000 to $34,999; 30 percent have access among those earning $35,000 to $49,999; and 52 percent of households with $50,000 or greater in income have an Internet connection. Barriers to Internet access include cost, lack of services in certain communities, limited literacy, lack of familiarity with different technologies, and, especially for people with disabilities, inaccessible formats that limit appropriate and effective technology use. Initiatives to promote universal access to the Internet will involve public and private sector stakeholders, particularly government agencies and technology corporations.

Potential data source: National Adult Literacy Survey,

2002, U.S. Department of Education. Responses from the National Adult Literacy Survey indicate that approximately 90 million adults in the United States have inadequate or marginal literacy skills. Written information is not the only way to communicate about health, but a great deal of health education and promotion are organised around the use of print materials, usually written at the 10th grade level and above. These materials are of little use to people who have limited literacy skills. The result is that a very large segment of the population is denied the full benefits of health information and services.

Closing the gap in health literacy is an issue of fundamental fairness and equity and is essential to reduce health disparities. Public and private efforts need to occur in two areas: the development of appropriate written materials and improvement in skills of those persons with limited literacy. The knowledge exists to create effective, culturally and linguistically appropriate, plain language health communications. Professional publications and Federal documents provide the criteria to integrate and apply the principles of organisation, writing style, layout, and design for effective communication. These criteria should be widely distributed and used. Many organisations such as public and medical libraries, voluntary, professional, and community groups, and schools could offer health literacy programmes that target skill improvement for low-literacy and limited English proficient individuals. If appropriate materials exist and people receive the training to use them, then measurable improvements in health literacy for the least literate can occur.

(Developmental) Increase the proportion of health communication activities that include research and evaluation.

Potential data sources: Sponsored survey of *Federal Register* notices; Grantmakers in Health; National Health Council.

Effective health communication programmes are built on sound research and evaluation. Meaningful research and evaluation are not afterthoughts but integral parts of initial programme design. Research provides the ideas and tools to design and carry out formative, process, and outcome evaluations to improve health communication efforts, certify the degree of change that has occurred, and identify programmes or elements of programmes that are not working. 10 Research and evaluation systematically obtain information that can be used to refine the design, development, implementation, adoption, redesign, and overall quality of a communication intervention. Programmes funded by Federal, philanthropic, and not-for-profit organisations could be strengthened with requirements for a minimum set of evaluation activities and specific measurements. The level of research and evaluation required should reflect the costs, scope, and potential impact (in terms of benefit or harm) of the communication activity proposed. At a minimum, programmes should be expected to conduct appropriate audience testing for need, cultural and linguistic competence, comprehension, and receptivity. Requirements and specifications for evaluation could be set for grant-funded communication programmes and included in requests for funding proposals and grant programme guidelines as well as for programmes directly funded and implemented by public or private sector organisations by including research and evaluation activities in their work plans.

(Developmental) Increase the proportion of health-related World Wide Web sites that disclose information that can be used to assess the quality of the site.

Potential data sources: Health on the Net Foundation; Health Internet Ethics (Hi-Ethics); Internet Healthcare Coalition.

With the rapidly growing volume of health information, advertising, products, and services available on World Wide Web sites, serious concerns arise regarding the accuracy, appropriateness, and potential health impact of these sites. People are using the Internet to look up information, purchase medications, consult remotely with providers, and maintain their personal health records. Approximately 70 million persons in the United States use the Internet for health-related reasons, and the potential for harm from inaccurate information, inferior quality goods, and inappropriate services is significant. Many initiatives are under way to identify appropriate and feasible approaches to evaluate online health sites. Professional associations are issuing guidelines and recommendations, Federal agencies such as the Federal Trade Commission are actively monitoring and sanctioning owners of Web sites that are false or misleading, and developers and purchasers of online health resources are being urged to adopt standards for quality assurance.

To allow users to evaluate the quality and appropriateness of Internet health resources, health-related Web sites should publicly disclose the following essential information about their site: (1) the identity of the developers and sponsors of the site (and how to contact them) and information about any potential conflicts of interest or biases, (2) the explicit purpose of the site, including any commercial purposes and advertising, (3) the original sources of the content on the site, (4) how the privacy and confidentiality of any personal information collected from users is protected, (5) how the site is evaluated, (6) and how the content is updated. An additional mark of quality which should be present in a Web site relates to the site's accessibility by all users. Contents of the site should be presented in a way that it can be used by people with disabilities and with low-end technology.

(Developmental) Increase the number of centers for excellence that seek to advance the research and practice of health communication.

Potential data sources: Health Communication Interest Group, American Public Health Association; Society for Social Marketing; Association of Schools of Public Health; Health Communication Divisions, International Communication Association and National Communication Association; NCI.

To enlarge the knowledge base of health communication and incorporate it into health promotion practice, a research and training infrastructure is needed to develop, model, and coordinate activities. For this purpose, centers for excellence located in academic institutions, national organisations, or research centers would be instrumental to meet scientific and practical needs. The centers would be responsible for an array of activities, such as (1) promoting the adoption of health communication theories and practices in health care, disease prevention, and health promotion initiatives, (2) developing and disseminating quality standards, (3) coordinating initiatives to develop a consensus research agenda, (4) developing systems to identify and assess health communication research, (5) evaluating communication strategies, messages, materials, and resources, (6) fostering networking and collaboration among health communicators, health educators, and other health professionals, (7) promoting health communication skills training for health professionals, and (8) promoting research and dissemination activities among specific population groups.

These centers should provide expert staff, model curricula with core competencies in health communication and media technologies, appropriately equipped media labs, research seminars, continuing education and distance learning courses, and training and placement programmes to expand the pool of health communication professionals and health professionals with communication skills. The centers also could create databases that would catalog items such as formative and outcomes research studies and reports and could partner with existing governmental dissemination networks to make data publicly available. Centers for excellence in health communication could be funded through Federal grants, foundations, or private sector health care organisations.

(Developmental) Increase the proportion of persons who report that their health care providers have satisfactory communication skills.

Potential data sources: National Committee for Quality Assurance; Behavioural Risk Factor Surveillance System (BRFSS), CDC, NCCDPHP; National Health Interview Survey (NHIS), CDC, NCHS; industry surveys (FIND/SVP, Nielsen, Jupiter Communications).

Good provider-patient communication contributes to quality care and improved health status. Patients' assessment of their providers' communication skills is important for individuals with a usual source of care as well as for those without, who may have less frequent contact with the medical care system. Studies indicate that patients find communicating with their health care providers difficult and report that providers do not give them enough information, even though they highly value the information and want to know more. Clear, candid, accurate, culturally and linguistically competent provider-patient communication is essential for the prevention, diagnosis, treatment, and management of health concerns.

Effective communication underpins prevention and screening efforts at the clinical level, when providers have the opportunity to engage in one-on-one counseling and supply information that is culturally and linguistically appropriate and delivered at the person's health literacy level. Diagnoses and treatments require doctors to negotiate a common understanding with patients about what is to be done. The quality of provider-patient communication can affect numerous outcomes, including patient adherence to recommendations and health status. Appropriate information and communication with a provider not only can relieve patients' anxieties but also can help patients understand their choices, allow them to participate in informed decisionmaking, and better manage their own health concerns.

5

Computer and Hospital Information Management System

CURRENT STATE OF COMPUTER TECHNOLOGY IN THE HEALTHCARE INDUSTRY

This chapter contains an examination of computer technology in the healthcare industry, from conceptual models to successfully operating applications demonstrating current or potential adaptations to healthcare, particularly in administrative functions. We also draw upon the results of surveys and focus groups to assess the readiness of New Jersey healthcare organisations for computerisation. The chapter ends with a brief discussion of the potential for computerisation of administrative functions in New Jersey.

Conceptual Models of the Healthcare Industry

Conceptual models of communication in the healthcare industry are in an advanced stage of development. Such models were proposed in the 1950s, with more advanced models being offered as recently as 1993. The following sections begin with a brief look at the major models developed since 1950 and conclude with an examination of a fully developed model derived from one segment of the healthcare industry, mental health.

The Seamless System Concept

Conceptual models range from integrated clinical and

fiscal management systems for mental health services [Newman and Sorenson, 1985] to comprehensive modeling of the entire healthcare industry as a "seamless system" of service delivery and communication in which the patient receives the right services from the right provider at the right time at reasonable cost [Wolford, Brown and McCool 1993]. An example of the seamless system of service appears in the integrated clinical and fiscal management system proposed by Newman and Sorenson on the basis of ten years of development involving operations and technology experts from across the United States. The purpose is to put client service and cost information together so managers can link the two in analyses to support management decisions [Newman and Sorenson, 1985, p. 281]. This method of application puts the focus on organisation management. The unconventional and expensive idea of computerizing clinical information gains credibility by enabling managers to analyse costs in the context of services delivered. These authors provide a step-by-step guidebook on how to develop such a system within an organisation such that all the required elements are compatible, linked with each other and relevant to the needs of clinical and managerial decision makers. In contrast, Wolford, Brown and McCool [1993, p. 9] propose a fully-integrated managed healthcare system at the "community" level:

> "...the ideal managed care delivery system will be an organised body of health services and financial mechanisms. It will operate in an integrated and systematic fashion to manage and provide the right wellness, medical and related services at the right place and time. The system's organisational goal will be to improve the long-term health status of the community.

Moreover, the ideal organisation will be designed to

function as a seamless system of services. Information will flow freely between the organised parts to provide a basis for customer convenience, provider and consumer learning, continuous improvement in delivery processes, avoidance of medical duplication, and containment of costs. Incentives will exist to focus the organised parts on the long-term improvement of community health status. The organised parts will be related through ownership and collaborative incentives to optimize the system versus optimizing the individual parts. Furthermore, mechanisms will be in place to assure community accountability and responsibility" [Wolford, Brown and McCool, 1993, p. 10]. Except for the fact that the authors explicitly state that their seamless system refers to an organisation incorporating both ownership and service delivery, [Wolford, Brown and McCool, p. 12], *their explication could refer to a communications system that permits the operating system to appear "seamless" to the consumers using it. But such a system need not be in an integrated organisation but can exist in the fragmented market system that Americans clearly prefer.* The HINT team believes that seamlessness can be accomplished by integrating communications using EDI and that this approach may allow Americans to retain their freedom to choose their providers of healthcare.

Early Models

Communication models for the healthcare industry were proposed as early as 1954 as a means of improving clinical practice and launched as early as 1966 as integrated, inter-sector, multi-unit systems [Glueck 1981]. The barriers to actual implementation of these conceptual models were money and technology. According to Glueck [1981, p. 7-8], his and other hospitals had adopted computers for many business tasks, but the idea of using computers for clinical information was unconventional and expensive. The researchers made some progress in a joint venture with a major insurance company, but the effort was stopped after two years because it was interfering with priority routine tasks on the hospital's overworked (mainframe) computers and had not generated any revenue-generating applications for the insurance company. *In 1981, technology constrained progress. Today, technology's capacity exceeds the will to apply it.*

Who Does What for Whom?

There are models characterizing healthcare as a paradigm: "Who does what for whom at what cost and with what effect?" [MHSIP 1989]. And, there are designs for minimum data sets supporting decision making at all levels, both within and among organisations. [MHSIP 1989]. The Mental Health Statistics Improvement Programme (MHSIP), a voluntary collaborative venture among the National Institute of Mental Health (NIMH), the National Association of State Mental Health Programme Directors (NASMHPD) and state mental health agencies, has as its goal enhancing the validity, reliability and comparability of mental health data to make it more useful to those who use it. Thus, the ability to freely exchange information is implied and the focus is on creating common understanding of the mental health system and achieving agreement on what data are important to stakeholders, that is, payers, providers, clinicians, patients, advocates, regulators and researchers. The efforts of MHSIP are relevant and important to the implementation of EDI because, as explained in Chapter 3, data standards and common formats are required for EDI implementation. One of the outputs of the MHSIP collaboration, Data Standards for Mental Health Decision Support Systems [1989], provides a rigorous comprehensive approach to, and minimum basic content of, data elements of systems for policy making, clinical care, management, evaluation and reporting. The data standards apply the paradigm (who does what to whom at what cost and with what effect?) to the information requirements in five domains. "Who" in the paradigm refers to those delivering the services, or the healthcare providers, both individual and organisational. "What" refers to the treatment or service "event" or "encounter", that is, to specify transactions with the healthcare provider. "Whom" refers to the person receiving services, i.e., in healthcare, the patient or client. Patient information includes personal information, medical history, symptoms, treatment plans, history and outcomes, insurance and payments. "At what cost" refers to the money required to provide services and constitutes the financial domain. "With what effect" measures the impact of services on the recipient's life and on society.

San Francisco Community Mental Health System

One of the uses of a multi-user information system with cost-saving potential is patient tracking [Nguyen 1987]. Developed as a "billing information system" (BIS) using mainframe computer technology, the San Francisco Community Mental Health System's billing information system lived up to its promise. The system was installed in 1981 in the over 100 separate agencies funded by the San Francisco System and used by those agencies to document service delivery to all patients. Their incentive to participate was the county's willingness to provide the computers and ensure access to current data and on the linkage of system utilisation to payment for services rendered. Money was the stick, expanded access to information the carrot. In the years from 1981-1987, the system increased Medicare collections twelve fold, doubled patient and insurance billings and increased Medi-Cal collections by 77 percent [Nguyen 1987, p. 1]. The per-dollar cost of collections fell from 16 cents to 10 cents during the time period. The patient-tracking system provided other important benefits as well. According to Nguyen [1987, p. 2-4], the system permits analysis of effort and performance, answering questions about the numbers and types of patients served, staff hours devoted to different types of patients, resources used by patient type and revenues generated or lost in serving various patients. The numbers and types of individual patients, it should be noted, is different from the number of events or encounters. When a system contains multiple providers and these providers report service utilisation, the reports contain events, not individuals. To track individuals in a data system, unique identifiers (e.g., SSN) must be assigned. The San Francisco system has such identifiers [Nguyen 1987, p. 4].

In addition to providing clinicians current information on a patient's medical history and recent service usage in other provider organisations, the multi-use system also permits analysis of clinical data about the treatment outcomes of specific patient groups, clinical status changes of groups of patients, tracking of the incidence and prevalence of illnesses and needs assessment. The information system also supports cost-benefit analyses of various treatments for patient groups and the level of status changes among groups of patients receiving different treatments. Finally, the system allows analysis of service utilisation patterns (type, intensity and duration) by diagnostic categories, demographic categories, providers and methods of treatment. The utilisation patterns of high users can be analysed as well. These applications are very important to the San Francisco system because it is the accountable public entity. The San Francisco system allocates and manages public funds to the over 100 public and private not-for-profit contractors. Thus, *the value of an integrated, multi-unit, multi-user information system goes beyond the billing needs of the single organisation or jurisdiction to become an important public management tool.*

Model Implications for Future Healthcare Information Systems

The focus of conceptual models, patient tracking and minimum data sets is improvement of service quality and cost effectiveness through access speed and timeliness, accuracy and comprehensiveness of information. The assumption is that service quality is improved because timely, accurate and comprehensive information facilitates more precise diagnosis and treatment; cost effectiveness is enhanced through improved service delivery and error reductions in documentation and reporting. This San Francisco System information system model operating since the early 1980s in a mental health delivery system is essentially the seamless system described for physical healthcare. It demonstrates more efficient delivery operations both by showing reduced administrative costs and increased revenue collections. Yet, it is not a single large monopolistic organisation as suggested by Wolford, Brown and McCool. Although based on a small geographical region, it incorporates multiple independent entities delivering a variety of services.

As the geographical region grows larger, and the technological capabilities of computers increase, the single computer network design used by the San Francisco system loses its appropriateness and multiple machine networks emerge as a required and desired option. However, the concept of integration of management information, including clinical information, into an accessible data base for multiple uses remains a dominant concept. In the following section, we describe current computer applications in two healthcare sectors likely to enjoy cost reductions from the application of EDI to administrative activities, that is, providers and payers.

Current Technological Applications

Substantial promise for administrative cost reductions through EDI utilisation for transaction activities such as claims submission, claims inquiry, payment advice, enrollment, and eligibility inquiry led the HINT team to identify computer technologies used for these activities. Applications in provider and payer sectors warrant description since these offer the greatest potential administrative efficiency improvement and cost reductions. It is not possible to describe all of the more than sixty sites visited during the process of examination. The HINT team appreciates the cooperation they received from all the sites and greatly appreciate the important insights provided by those in various stages of implementing computer technologies. Each and every site visited enriched the team's knowledge and understanding. The selection of two sectors for inclusion in this report is, therefore, somewhat arbitrary. The described sectors' providers and payers activities represent advanced technological applications with clear concern for electronic communication. Our description of these applications is greatly enriched by the input of all cooperating sites; and we are most grateful for that input.

Providers and payers are the healthcare entities involved in administrative activities with the greatest potential for increased efficiency and cost reductions through EDI. Among providers, we focus on hospitals primarily because, as large organisational units, hospitals tend to be more advanced in their application of computers. Among payers, the focus is one traditional indemnity insurer, an HMO, and an intermediary, i.e., a claims processor, all of whom have implemented electronic information transfer at some level.

Providers - Hospitals

Hospitals are the traditional core of the healthcare system in New Jersey. As large organisations with a noticeable physical presence and a history of community service, hospitals are integral to a community, both as service providers and as symbols of the community's public service image. Hospitals vary widely in the degree of computerisation used in delivering healthcare services and managing their operations. Computerisation ranges from simple accounting and billing operations to extensive computerisation including pharmaceutical dispensing at nursing stations. To capture the sense of this range of computer technology application, the HINT team visited several hospitals in various states of computerisation. Herein we report on three which help to shed light on the local climate for computerisation of transaction activities using EDI. The hospitals are Columbia-Presbyterian Medical Center in New York City, Atlantic City Medical Center and St. Joseph's Hospital in Patterson. Each is addressed in turn.

Columbia-Presbyterian Medical Center

Columbia Presbyterian Medical Center (CPMC) is located in New York City just across the George Washington Bridge from New Jersey. Thus, it is virtually a "local" hospital for New Jersey. CPMC is a university teaching hospital, one of 358 in the United States in 1986 [Kovner 1990, p. 148]. Teaching hospitals are larger than most hospitals and usually are located in large metropolitan areas. They offer many specialized services and provide significant amounts of uncompensated care. In 1986, over half of the national Council of Teaching Hospital members averaged six times the outpatient visits and over four times the surgeries of other hospitals [Kovner 1990, p. 148]. Teaching hospitals tend to be more capital intensive than non-teaching hospitals. For example, in 1986, 87 percent of these hospitals reported having a cardiac catheterisation lab as compared to 16 percent of other hospitals, and 45 percent of teaching hospitals reported the ability to do organ transplants, compared to 3 percent of other hospitals [Kovner 1990, p. 148]. Regarding charity care, in 1985, teaching hospitals had 20 percent of all short-term beds but 30 percent of the Medicaid bad debts and charity care. These hospitals represented 6 percent of all non-federal hospitals in 1984, but claimed 49 percent of total deductions for charity care and 36 percent of the deductions for bad debt [Kovner 1990, p. 148].

Columbia-Presbyterian Medical Center is a typical, complex teaching hospital. Situated in a medically under served community in northern Manhattan [Hendrickson, et.al. 1992]. CPMC consists of a number of institutions, each with its own administration and governing body. The Columbia University portion of the medical center is headed by a vice president for health sciences who reports to the president. The Presbyterian Hospital is a 1500 bed not-for-profit hospital located in the medical complex. Presbyterian recently opened the Allen Pavilion, a 300-bed community hospital three miles north, and operates a network of ambulatory clinics in northern Manhattan. The New York State Psychiatric Institute also is part of the medical center, as is the Health Sciences Library, funded by Columbia University.

The effort to introduce EDI in this complex system characterized by many highly specialized participants with varied needs required the same kind of coordination that will be required to establish EDI across sectors of the fragmented healthcare industry. The approach taken by CPMC combined high-placed committed leadership with a non-hierarchical approach to development. That is, participants needed to "buy into" the common network and workstation architecture, but once on the system they could develop whatever applications they wished [Hendrickson, et.al. 1992, p. 39]. Early development of policies on issues of data ownership, data confidentiality and data integrity, and stringent controls on access to sensitive information like student records, payroll information and clinical data facilitated acceptance [Hendrickson, et.al. 1992, p. 39].

The implemented EDI system at CPMC permits authorized user access to seven functions. These functions range from core services like network, e-mail and basic communications to a variety of information and research services [Hendrickson, et. al. 1992, p. 36]. Among the information services are clinical information (medical records, order entry and nursing), administrative services (space and facilities, directories, grants management, personnel, word processing, desktop publishing) and scholarly information services (library, electronic textbook, natural language processing). Among the research services are clinical research services (epidemiology, research databases, statistical packages) and basic medical research (biomedical research tools, super-computing and graphics). Finally, medical informatics research provides operations support and access to decision making, knowledge base, workstations, human interface and education. The CPMC integrated information system is an example of efficient communication wherein data is entered into the system only once and it is developed into information often and in varied ways. The system uses a large mainframe as its core for integrated communication among its widely dispersed user groups. In addition, the mainframe includes a link to the Internet international communication network. This allows authorized users to enter the system from any location in the world and obtain information. This was demonstrated when a CPMC authorized user visited NJIT's Newark Campus in September, 1993. Using an NJIT work station and NJIT's Internet connection, the authorized user connected with CPMC's mainframe and obtained information on several of his patients. CPMC uses the "Health Level Seven" (HL-7) standard application communication protocol discussed in detail in Chapter 3. This protocol allows proprietary systems to communicate with each other on a one-to-one basis regardless of the language used in each individual system. HL-7 is a "translator" protocol that represents a major step forward in computer communication between dissimilar hardware/software systems. CPMC has been a leader in its application and promotion. The Internet link on CPMC's mainframe computer system demonstrates that a high speed mainframe intra-hospital communication system can be linked into EDI applications even though the system is a proprietary system. Over the longer term, CPMC hopes to provide access to its sophisticated medical image electronic communication system to outsiders over the external EDI connection.

Atlantic City Medical Center, NJ

Atlantic City Medical Center belongs to the category of multi-hospital system because it consists of two or more hospitals either under contract management or legally incorporated by or under the direction of a single board [Kovner 1990, p. 148]. In 1986, 44 percent, or 278, of the nation's hospitals were multi-hospital systems consisting of 2,514 hospitals and 429,837 beds [Kovner 1990, p. 149]. Large multi-hospital systems frequently own other types of providers as well, for example, nursing homes, psychiatric hospitals, retirement centers, home healthcare and management contract businesses. Ownership of multi-hospital systems may be public, private or private not-for-profit. Private for-profit systems are large, averaging 23 hospitals spread over many states [Kovner 1990, p. 149]. Private not-for-profit multi-hospital systems tend to be small, averaging seven hospitals per system located in one or a few contiguous states. Among public hospital systems, the Veterans Administration, with over 160 hospitals, and the

New York City Health and Hospitals Corporation, with 11 hospitals, are notable. Atlantic City Medical Center is a two-hospital system. Its second hospital is located in Pomona, NJ. Because of the distance between the two facilities and the need for transfer of patients and information between the two, Atlantic City Medical Center is vitally aware of the problems of inter-facility communication.

For this reason, the Center's systems development group designed its computerisation plan around a translator computer, that is, a computer capable of speaking with all proprietary systems in the "vocabulary and language" of each. This translator computer is called a "gateway or interface engine." The interface engine will have the ability to receive a communication from one proprietary system, translate it into the language of a second proprietary system and complete the communication to the second system. The interface engine is basically a translation device. The design assumes that most communications will use Health Level Seven as the standard protocol. The long term objective of the overall system is to connect all major functions in the hospitals with each other thereby supporting a case management system allowing direct physician order entry and results reporting through computer commands. Currently, financial, laboratory, cardiology, pharmacy and medical record abstract systems are computerized with proprietary hardware and software. At the time of the interview, the interface engine was not yet installed. The interface engine design is one technological approach to overcoming the barrier of incompatibility of proprietary systems. In an ideal world, each proprietary system would have an output device that would communicate in a standard language to any system outside itself. If all proprietary systems used the same standard language, then all systems could communicate with all others. In the real world, interface engines are necessary components of any design to produce an integrated hospital information system from among different subsystems.

When asked about a connection to an EDI system, the Director of the ACMC systems development group replied that the interface engine can be programmed to connect to a network and communicate in whatever standard protocol the network requires. Thus, the ACMC interface engine design is flexible and will accommodate EDI when EDI becomes available.

St. Joseph's Hospital, Patterson, NJ

St. Joseph's Hospital in Patterson, New Jersey is a community hospital. Community hospitals are non-federal short-term general or specialty hospitals (except psychiatric, tuberculosis and respiratory disease hospitals) that serve the public [Kovner 1990, p. 145]. Community hospitals come in many sizes, ranging from small rural hospitals under 50 beds to large hospitals over 500 beds. St. Joseph's is a mid-sized hospital. The large majority (75 percent) of community hospitals are owned by private not-for-profit corporations. Most community hospitals offer a range of services to the communities they serve and are valued members of their communities. Typically, community hospitals offer general medical and surgical care in inpatient and outpatient settings, diagnostic tests, emergency services, intensive care services, preventive services, and one or more specialty services. St. Joseph's Hospital recently acquired a new computerized information system. An entirely new system was acquired because the old (legacy) systems were not adequate for upgrading. St. Joseph's had been using a contractor for computerized claims processing and financial reports but decided to have the contractor install a complete clinical and administrative system under an eight year contract. The new system began operating in

April, 1994, with over 2,000 people being retrained, including doctors, nurses, clerical personnel and other users during the 18 months preceding the April startup.

The new system consists of integrating separate functions into a single, large computer to minimize communication problems. Simply stated, the large machine can talk to itself without problems of language or transmission protocols. However, some specialized proprietary systems remain disconnected from the network, such as magnetic resonance imaging machines and x-ray machines. St. Joseph's computerized information system represents the most current in applied main frame computer technology. Yet, it is not set up for electronic data interchange through a network. The designers of the system do not foresee the early advent of an EDI network and therefore saw no reason to include a connection in their system. With the addition of the earlier described translation technologies, the St. Joseph system can, however, be modified to accommodate EDI connections in the future.

Payers - Insurers and HMOs

In addition to site visits to providers, the HINT team visited major indemnity insurers and HMOs. The team also visited New Jersey based claims processing companies. While not payers in the strict sense, claims processors have an integral role in the administrative function's transaction activities. The team describes herein three organisations representing EDI thinking and actions among payers.

Prudential Insurance Company

The Prudential Insurance Company is a private, broad product line indemnity insurer offering healthcare insurance as one of many types of insurance products. The tradition of such indemnity insurance is to charge employers or individuals annual premiums and pay healthcare providers on a fee-for-service basis [Kovner 1990, p. 282]. Prudential also contracts "administrative services only" with self-insured companies, for example AT&T. "Administrative services only" means that Prudential has no financial risk for AT&T employees but provides healthcare claims processing. Upon claims adjudication, Prudential makes the payment on behalf of the employer or commits the employer to make the payment. This latter line of work, administrative services or third party administrators (TPAs), is one of the most rapidly growing areas of healthcare payment today. Administrative services is particularly relevant to HINT's interests because it requires more communication between the insurance company and the employer since the TPA not only needs the name of the benefits subscriber but also needs to report subscriber benefit payments back to the employer.

The mass of inter-organisational communication between Prudential and AT&T required by the administrative services contract with AT&T led Prudential to participate in the development of an EDI employee enrollment system during 1993. This system uses Health Care Financing Administration (HCFA) standard formats and transmission protocols described in Chapter 3. The system allows AT&T's personnel department to enroll employees on Prudential's computers with no transmission of paper. The system is described in detail in Chapter 4, and it is currently *operating with savings to both Prudential and AT&T*. Since this successful EDI application was initiated, Prudential has offered it to other employers throughout the United States. Because the system is built upon HCFA standards, it can be implemented as part of contract payment services, indemnity insurance or HMO enrollments, all of which can be transmitted on open networks.

US Healthcare

US Healthcare is an independent practice association (IPA) model health maintenance organisation in which the HMO (US Healthcare) contracts with independent physicians and groups to provide healthcare services to HMO members [Kovner 1990, p. 256]. IPA model HMOs are characterized by the need to manage service utilisation and contain costs in a decentralized service distribution network. EDI is an appropriate technology for such a network. US Healthcare is one of the fastest growing HMOs in the U.S. and especially New Jersey. US Healthcare has adopted the "capitation" form of physician payment, i.e., it pays a physician a flat fee for all the healthcare services delivered to each patient during a specific period of time. However, US Healthcare requires physicians to file "encounter reports" to document each encounter with a patient. These encounter reports are as numerous as are claims in the fee for service delivery systems.

To reduce the work required to submit, receive and review encounter reports, US Healthcare encourages physicians to use computerized reporting. To facilitate electronic communications, US Healthcare acquired Orion Computer Systems, Inc., a supplier of physician office practice computer systems. Orion includes with its system an electronic link to US Healthcare's computers so that the physician can file encounter reports, and referrals directly from its computer to US Healthcare computers. In return, the physician can use the electronic link to obtain information from US Healthcare on patient demographics, eligibility and benefits; hospital admissions and discharges; specialists directory; procedures directory; capitation summaries; and responses to inquiries (e-mail). In addition, the Orion physician practice system allows physicians to file claims electronically with other claims processing organisations by directing the communication to the claims processor's computer.

Clearly, US Healthcare has identified the cost saving potential of electronic communication and has established itself as a supplier of both ends of the communication system. However, it encourages its providers to use a proprietary system, useful primarily to US Healthcare and its contract providers although it can be adapted to submit claims to claims processors. The Orion system does not offer an open network nor does the data travel on an open network. Electronic connections are made via telephone lines directly to US Healthcare's computers (or a claims processor's computers). Thus, in its present form, the Orion system is a terminal type system wherein the physician's computer becomes a terminal communicating directly with US Healthcare's computer. The system is therefore primarily proprietary to US Healthcare. In its present form, this EDI system does not generate a data flow that is accessible to government analysts nor public policy researchers. On the other hand, *US Healthcare's actions make clear that the benefits of computer transmission of encounter reports are real, not imaginary.*

National Electronic Information Corporation

National Electronic Information Corporation (NEIC), a Secaucus, New Jersey headquartered company is one of the largest electronic healthcare transaction networks in the nation. It has 14 years of experience in the electronic healthcare transaction business and represents a very advanced electronic communications system. Although many providers refer to is as a "claims clearinghouse," it provides a variety of electronic communications services for hospitals, medical and dental providers directly and through contracts with 87 computer system vendors and clearinghouses doing business in New Jersey. Such communications include claims, encounter reports, eligibility and plan benefit information, electronic remittance advice, claims status reports, and other reports.

Providers willingly pay for NEIC's specialized services since it relieves the provider from the highly specialized burden of communicating with a variety of healthcare organisations whose computers operate with many different languages. NEIC does this by providing computer to computer communication in the language of the organisation with which it is communicating.. In this way, NEIC operates much like a EDI network, except that it must accommodate, or translate, a variety of language standards from different organisations. For example, NEIC can connect a New Jersey hospital's computer to a Connecticut payer's computer even though the communication, such as a claim form, is received from the hospital in one format and protocol and transmitted to the payer in another format and protocol. NEIC provides communication with over 71 payers in New Jersey and nationwide. However, since there are over 450 different payer claim forms [Cook, 1993], and NEIC does not handle all of these, providers still have to file some claims manually. Nonetheless, *NEIC is as close to an open EDI network as present technology and lack of standards will allow.*

Payer Summary

The healthcare third party payment process has changed considerably with the emergence of numerous different insurers, administrative services contractors, HMOs, and PPOs. This proliferation of payment methods has greatly increased the variety and complexity of the payment process, and expanded the complexity of the communications required. Nonetheless, claims remain the basic mechanism for provider collection of fees in a fee-for-service system The proliferation of payers makes claims submission so complex that specialists in this task have emerged to assist providers with this task. NEIC is one of many private organisations operating around the country that make a profit by reducing the cost of communication of claims for both the provider and payer. Claims are replaced by "encounter reports" in HMOs using capitation payment systems because, although no payment transfers are involved in a capitation system, the HMOs want information about who does what to whom. Without reporting of information about what services are provided under what conditions, HMO payers are without the information they need for planning and control.

Both the existing computer communications systems and the HMO's have taken important steps towards reducing administrative costs. But none of these have achieved the level of administrative cost reduction that can be attained with a fully operational, EDI open network. And, the current state of the healthcare industry does not provide adequate incentives for the development and operation of an EDI open network. Computer communications technology has advanced as far as it can given the absence of standards. The Prudential/AT&T adoption of a standard form and standard published transmission protocol for use on an open network to enroll employees is a singular, but notable step towards adoption of EDI in New Jersey.

Information Providers - MedE America, Inc.

Neither a payer nor a provider, MedE America is another independent business providing administrative transaction-related services for healthcare providers, particularly hospitals. Its service is electronic eligibility verification via on-line information. This service addresses a major problem in urban hospitals which is determining whether patients have healthcare coverage. Some patients misrepresent themselves as indigent and uninsured to avoid paying deductible or co-pay amounts. Others are indigent, may be eligible for Medicaid, but are unaware or never have applied.

The hospital can assist the Medicaid eligible patient to apply at the time of healthcare service delivery and assure the hospital's reimbursement. What the hospital needs, and MedE America provides, is patient identification verification combined with systematic, reliable, eligibility verification.

MedE America fulfills the eligibility verification part of the hospital's needs by providing a computerized system to determine patient eligibility for healthcare benefits. MedE America's system has access agreements with a large number of payers, including New York State Medicaid, and offers on-line electronic inquiry into patient eligibility for payment from these payers. MedE America's system is widely used in New York State where it has special legislative authorisation to operate. Its service for unambiguous patient identification consists of verification of patient addresses to assure that the patient has given correct address information during admission. This is less verification than hospitals desire but better than anything else available. Initially, MedE America's service was a telephone inquiry/ response system. But, it is converting into a full EDI system with 50 hospitals connected through terminals by the end of 1994. MedE America sells its service at a profit. The service is not inexpensive but 35 percent of the hospitals in New York find that their increased revenues justify the costs for services delivered by MedE America.

Community Health Management Information System (CHMIS)

Since 1990, the John A. Hartford Foundation has actively funded and promoted the concept of community health management information systems (CHMIS). The first pilot projects began operation in 1991 and since then Hartford Foundation money has supported CHMIS development in Iowa, Minnesota, New York, Ohio, Memphis, Tennessee,

Vermont, and Washington state.

In the Hartford design, CHMIS consists of three elements:

A communications network;

Standard transactions that flow on the network;

A data repository of network information.

The communications network is defined as an open network with published standards that allow any user whose hardware and software meet the standards and has authorisation to connect and use the system. This means that any participant in the healthcare industry can connect to the network and transmit and receive information. The standard transactions are defined with published standards so that any user can implement the transactions with appropriate hardware/software that meets the standards. Thus, any participant can transmit any transaction to any other participant. This element ensures that the network is open. The data repository is a data base that accumulates and stores information flowing across the network. The repository can be used by authorized users to develop patient profiles, provider profiles, payer profiles, and community profiles. Such profiles can be used for government-approved payer and provider evaluations as well as community health monitoring. In addition, policy and medical research can be carried out with such a data base. A nearby installation of a CHMIS funded in part by the Hartford Foundation is the New York State CHMIS. Currently, the Hartford Foundation is not funding any additional CHMIS development efforts. However, its experiences in a variety of settings makes it a excellent source of information for implementation of a healthcare EDI network.

Summary of Current Applications

As is apparent from the array of applications presented

above, *EDI exists in bits and pieces around the nation, in well-developed concepts and specialized commercial applications by a variety of suppliers.* We have described typical examples of leading edge technological applications. These "bits and pieces", when combined in a conceptualisation and comprehensive implementation such as CHMIS, provide a framework, of necessary elements and methods for applying computer technology to reduce administrative costs. Technology leaders have identified the destination and are providing the road maps, but the trip is barely started. Two essential elements, the networks and standard transactions, are operationalized in individual applications, but have not been implemented widely. The data repository concept needs development. The Hartford Foundation is currently funding a major study by the RAND Corporation designed to establish clear standards for the structure and data elements of a repository. Given the experience of data standards development in the mental health system, development of healthcare medical data standards will be a slow process. And, development is not acceptance and implementation. These, like implementation of networks and standardized transactions, may be problematic. If the technology is so obvious and applied in bits and pieces, one might ask, why is there no rush to adopt EDI? The barriers are considered next.

Barriers To Adoption of EDI in New Jersey

WEDI addressed the issue of barriers to adoption of EDI and summarized its findings in the following way:

"Compared with other industries such as financial services, retail, and manufacturing, the "business information" exchanged in healthcare is widely considered to be more complex and variable. This complexity has inhibited the development and adoption of standards that would enable widespread automation of healthcare business interactions. For example, it is estimated that only 15% of the 4.8 billion annual healthcare claims are currently submitted electronically and the percentage of other healthcare transactions handled electronically is insignificant (i.e., less than one percent). The relative lack of electronic communication in healthcare today creates a tremendous opportunity for significant administrative and clinical cost savings if comprehensive, standardized EDI capabilities are adopted throughout the industry" [WEDI, 1993, p. 9-11].

A nationwide survey of healthcare industry participants conducted by the WEDI group in 1992 elicited reasons for the reluctance to adopt EDI [WEDI, 1992, Appendix 8, pp. 1-5]. Similar questions were asked of New Jersey healthcare industry participants in the HINT mail survey conducted by TESC's HINT socio/economic team in early 1994. Focus groups conducted in 1994 also considered this subject. The results of these three inquiries are reported below.

WEDI 1992 Survey

The WEDI survey of over 2200 healthcare providers, payers, technology vendors, employers, consumers and lawyers was designed to identify, among other things, major obstacles to achieving electronic data interchange of information in the healthcare industry. WEDI identified twelve perceived obstacles, which the group rank ordered [WEDI, 1992, Appendix 2, p. iii]:

- Lack of standard data sets, definitions or formats;
- Lack of recognised national standard-setting authority;
- Complexity of healthcare delivery and health insurance process;
- Costs associated with conversion, installation and maintenance;

— Confidentiality concerns;
— Lack of effective communications;
— Legal/regulatory barriers;
— Resistance to change;
— Lack of Incentives;
— Lack of belief that uniform EDI will happen;
— Lack of national directory of healthcare providers and payers;
— Lack of cooperation among the participants.

These obstacles are expressed from the viewpoints of individual participants' specific organisational perspectives of conditions that require inter-organisational actions as the preceding examples of applications show. In other words, individuals are very pessimistic about system-wide change.

Explanation of WEDI Obstacles

The lack of standard data elements or data set definitions or formats prevents the transfer of data from one computer to another because no computer system can interpret or understand incoming data that arrives in an unknown format. This is a technical barrier that has been solved in private sector industries because appropriate incentives (profits) are in place. WEDI survey respondents perceive that no common basis for electronic communication among sectors in the healthcare industry exists, so EDI is not possible. The proliferation of EDI usage in the private sector proves the technological capability and inter-organisational benefits of EDI. And there are both comprehensive conceptual and specifically defined minimum data sets and standards available in healthcare. Thus, this is a perceived technical barrier caused by an incentives problem. The profit incentive is, in fact, beginning to solve the problem in the healthcare industry, because businesses are forming to provide EDI linkages. However, this is not efficient from the healthcare system perspective because these applications are partial, have not adopted uniform standards, and do not remove the systemic complexities. For example, 450 different claims forms asking for similar data in separate formats still exist and this complexity cannot be resolved by those firms providing limited EDI services.

There is no recognised standard-setting authority to establish standards. This is no surprise given the fragmented nature of the industry. As explained in Chapter 1, no single healthcare sector participant dominates the industry and, because the financial goals of sectors are conflicting, no participant has the incentive to resolve the communications problems of the others, even though the solution would benefit all participants. Currently, the decision about standards is individual and proprietary. That is, a sector participant buys a particular computer system and with it, the standards set by the manufacturer. For EDI, as the Columbia-Presbyterian Medical Center example shows, each participant must agree to a common network and workstation (or communications) architecture. To achieve such common communications capability throughout the industry with a single proprietary system is to have a monopoly. That is, if a single company were to sell so many of its own systems that its system becomes the standard, the proprietary system captures the market and becomes a monopoly, with all its attendant problems, including the ability to manipulate price. Not a good outcome, the HINT team argues. On the other hand, given the conflicting goals of particular industry sectors (payers and providers) and the competitiveness of within sector participants (either payers or providers), there is no incentive for one or a few participants to come together voluntarily to establish standards and then try to persuade its communication partners to adopt this same standard for themselves and all their communication partners. That involves high costs with few visible benefits accruing to the initiators of such a system. Indeed, the optimum decision for any user in the industry is do nothing unless or until a meaningful industry-wide standard emerges. Thus, there is no market incentive except monopoly market power for an authority to exist and no incentive for sector participants to create such an authority.

These perceptions cause healthcare industry participants to become negative about the future of EDI and express this in obstacle number 10, *lack of belief that EDI will happen*. The participants simply do not see a standard setting organisation in existence and recognise that voluntary standards adoption is most unlikely. The third obstacle is the *complexity of the healthcare delivery process and insurance system*. With over 3000 payers and over 450 different claim forms, with rapidly increasing numbers of independent providers, with new and frequently changing regulatory requirements and service documentation, the US healthcare system is indeed complex. But, as previous discussions and technical material in subsequent chapters makes clear, many complexities can be simplified through widespread implementation of EDI computer technology. Thus, this is a perceived obstacle that will dissipate as EDI becomes the communications technology of the healthcare industry.

Cost of converting to EDI is the fourth obstacle perceived by respondents to the WEDI survey. This obstacle must be considered in the context of the one before it. That is, conversion costs are problematic without standards to facilitate EDI adoption by all participants. Once standards are set, EDI adoption becomes attractive to all sectors. As shown in Chapter 3, the cost of hardware and software requirements for EDI will be relatively small since technology costs are falling rapidly. The major costs are training costs. These can be considerable, especially for the small provider with only one or two administrative personnel. Additional incentives may be necessary to speed up adoption by some participants.

Confidentiality of data emerges as the fifth obstacle. The information privacy right is important to consumers and providers. As discussed in Chapter 3, EDI is an open system with large amounts of patient information available in a single place with immense search and retrieve capability. The concern is that unauthorized persons may gain access and once into the system, easily obtain data on a large number of patients. In the CHMIS example described earlier, a key element of adoption was early agreement to policies on confidentiality and related issues about data: ownership, integrity and access controls. Such policies, and effective monitoring systems, will be necessary if EDI is to be successfully applied to achieve administrative cost reductions in the healthcare industry.

The lack of communications refers to the technical incompatibility among communications partners and the proliferation of communications documents already mentioned. Thus, in the perceptions of respondents, it is a technical barrier partly caused by the complexity of the industry and the lack of standards. Thus, this perceived barrier also reflects the lack of incentives for individual participants to seek system solutions. In the meantime, proprietary suppliers of hardware and software to the healthcare industry continue to seek competitive advantage by convincing payers and providers to adopt EDI, one by one. As noted above, however, proprietary technology is designed to function and interact with a set of standards that are unique to a specific supplier. Adopting one supplier's hardware commits the user to acquiring all future software from vendors that write software for that specific piece of hardware. Such software is unlikely to be useful with any other supplier's hardware. Differences in hardware and software among suppliers means that communications among them are difficult at best. Thus, a hardware purchase decision commits the buyer to a long period of dependency on a single supplier. The supplier is happy about this, but, given the goal of cost reductions and the nature of monopolies in market economies, it would not be a good outcome for the industry.

The *existence of contractual, legal and regulatory barriers* contains two reference points. One is related to complexity and duplication, the other to legal constraints against collusion.

Regarding complexity and duplication, for example, New Jersey requires DRG reports that contain much of the same information as insurance claim forms, but the DRG reports must be filed in a different way with a different format from insurance claims. Insurance companies vary in the type of information they want on a claim form and the extent to which they want documents attached to claim forms. These complexities have led to the development of market mechanisms to simplify the process for providers. For example many existing electronic communications systems serving the healthcare industry carry claims to a large but not exhaustive list of payers. Subscribers to one of these systems must also subscribe to another claims submitting system or submit claims manually to the remaining payers. These responses do nothing to remove the systemic problems of duplication of filing that may be required by state or local reports, such as the DRGs in New Jersey. Regarding legal constraints, healthcare participants are subject to antitrust laws limiting interactions that may be construed as interfering with market forces. For example, if insurers were to initiate an effort to standardize claims reporting forms, they could be accused of anti-trust violations, much as institutions of higher education were accused and later exonerated of "price fixing" a few years back because they worked together on student financial aid packages. The potential legal costs of even erroneous charges successfully prevent a decision to cooperate, thereby making a cooperative effort involving industry participants, such as the WEDI group, impossible without government sponsorship. This also is the substance of obstacle twelve, *a lack of cooperation among the participants*.

Resistance to change is a common intra-organisational problem, but when combined with the absence of *incentives to change* as reflected in barrier number nine, becomes an unyielding block. The healthcare industry, therefore, is caught in a trap of rigid, inefficient, administrative operations over which individual participants have little control and no incentives to change. It is little wonder that those without an appreciation for the power of unleashed technology can see only vertical integration of functions as an option. Their response is to put the incentives for change in an organisational hierarchy incorporating payer and provider in hopes of accomplishing savings not otherwise possible. Their assumption is that the claims processing tasks will be eliminated to save costs. Given the need for cost analysis and other management information, however, the elimination of claims processing will not mean the elimination either of documentation and reporting or of routine inter-organisational communications.

If the tasks will remain, it is essential to provide incentives to be efficient in carrying out those tasks. If the task is essentially inter-organisational, the incentives must be external to separate participants but common to the industry. Obstacle eleven recognises another technical requirement of EDI, *the need for a comprehensive list of healthcare providers and payers*. Participants must be able to locate one another if EDI, or any communication linkage is to be possible. There are lists of providers and payers as close as the local phone book or directory assistance and comprehensive lists in a variety of locations. For example, departments of insurance maintain lists of insurers operating in the state and membership associations keep membership current lists. Likewise, state licensing departments will have rosters of those licensed to operate. However, because these lists are specialized and kept by separate organisations, there can be substantial search costs in identification. Also, lists may be neither exhaustive nor current. To make EDI work for everyone, all participants in relevant sectors need to be identified by unique identifiers and addresses. While this may appear to be a significant barrier to individual participants, once the incentives for broad-based communications are in place, it is technically resolved rather easily.

Clearly, technology exists to overcome technical barriers, and standards exist to establish a fully operational EDI system for the healthcare industry. On the other hand, the competitive environment among providers, payers and technology suppliers will not go away, nor should we want it to. Neither will the conflicting goals between payers and providers dissipate. Legal constraints will continue to prevent a mood of cooperation among payers unless that mood is stimulated by a neutral force, as happened when the federal government encouraged formation of WEDI. WEDI, in turn, strongly recommends government action to establish EDI standards for the healthcare industry [WEDI, 1993, p. 6]

Barriers to EDI Adoption in New Jersey

Using WEDI's findings as a model for its inquiry, the HINT team examined New Jersey healthcare participants' perceptions and experiences about the current and potential use of EDI for administrative tasks in New Jersey. The two techniques used were focus groups and a mail survey, the details of which appear in the socio-economic team's report.

Both the mail survey and focus groups were designed to obtain information from participants in all healthcare sectors:

— Hospitals; claims processing and medical records
— Physicians;
— Medical and radiology laboratories;
— Pharmacies;
— Insurance companies, HMOs and third party administrators.

The mail survey contained factual questions about current computer use and its attendant costs with some additional questions regarding respondent intentions for expanded use of computers. Focus groups were designed to elicit information on the extent of computer use and attitudes towards expanding computer use. In the following section, we draw from these two sources information relevant to identification of barriers to adoption of computerisation in general and EDI in particular.

Survey Responses

Mail survey responses show that 86 percent of hospitals, 33 percent of physicians, 40 percent of laboratories, and 89 percent of pharmacies use computers. With the exception of pharmacies, the vast majority of computer applications are proprietary systems used solely for internal operations. Pharmacies use EDI systems to communicate with suppliers and maintain patient records. Eighty-one percent of the hospitals responding use computers for claims processing; however, claims are submitted on data tapes, not electronically using EDI. Hospitals also continue to file many claims manually. Thus, hospitals are knowledgeable in the use of computers for administrative activities and are aware of the administrative efficiencies gained from submitting claims electronically rather than by paper form. Laboratories and physicians use computers primarily for administrative tasks as well.

One survey question asked about the importance of factors influencing a decision to acquire a computerized system. There are four factors, presented here in order of their importance to respondents:

— Costs
— Quality of care
— Convenience/usability
— Individual preferences.

New Jersey respondents rank costs most important. Cost factors are time-efficiency, cost of hardware and cost-efficiency. All sectors rate cost factors most important, but physicians give cost factors higher average importance than other factors. Since the New Jersey survey did not focus specifically on EDI, but rather on computerisation in general, the concern about cost clearly is a direct statement about immediate organisational realities, not a relative statement, as was the cost statement in the WEDI survey. The number one ranking reflects the degree to which cost concerns have come to permeate healthcare sector participants' operating decisions. The importance of cost concerns, earlier reported comments of individuals during HINT team site visits to New Jersey entities and the systemic incentive problems described elsewhere in this chapter, combine to suggest that EDI could not be cost justified at this time.

Quality of care consists of two dimensions: improving healthcare delivery and confidentiality. Improving healthcare delivery ranked second among all sectors but was given higher average scores by hospitals' medical records respondents and pharmacies. Confidentiality issues are a lesser quality concern to respondents than improving healthcare delivery quality. One might argue that the low level of concern about confidentiality occurs because respondents are thinking about intra-organisational, single use computer systems. However, among this survey's respondents, pharmacies, whose computer systems are inter-organisational, give confidentiality concerns a lower average score than other sectors. As noted earlier, on the national survey on EDI, confidentiality ranked fifth among the twelve identified concerns. How New Jersey healthcare industry participants would view confidentiality relative to EDI is, therefore, not clear from these results. Five convenience/usability factors are considered. The transition of existing records is listed by all sectors as the most important convenience/usability factor affecting the decision to computerize. The decision to computerize entails related decisions, one of which is what to do about historical records. Some computer systems may require entering large amounts of historical data before the system can be operational. Other systems can be started up as of a certain date without regard to historical information. Systems requiring initial data input are more costly and inconvenient. Thus, it is not surprising that physicians, for whom historical information is critical to current operations, gave this a higher score than other sectors. This issue was not raised in the WEDI national survey.

Availability of standard format or codes is an important convenience/usability factor as well, and closely parallels the greatest concern expressed in the national survey, that is, the lack of standard data sets, formats or codes. Among New Jersey respondents, physicians and hospitals give this higher scores than do labs and pharmacies. The elaborate coding required for documentation of healthcare service delivery is the likely source of importance of this dimension to physicians and hospitals. The importance of standard formats to EDI has already been discussed.

The complexity of technology and additional training required are also convenience/usability dimensions and are ranked third and fourth among these dimensions. Physicians rank these higher on average than the other sector participants. Since physicians are also the least likely to be using computers currently (33 percent). It is probable that they are less computer literate. This means training costs will be added to purchase and installation costs for any computer adoptions by physicians, raising the average costs of computerisation for physicians. The concern and associated costs, therefore, are likely to affect EDI adoption as well. Individual preference factors, specifically physicians' preferences and preferences of other personnel or customers, ranked last and, overall, were given low scores by all participants. Thus, their impact on the likelihood of computerisation is negligible. The results of this New Jersey survey are not directly comparable to the WEDI survey. New Jersey providers have more concerns about costs of computerisation and its ability to improve service delivery and less concern about confidentiality and technical considerations. Costs and quality of healthcare service delivery are therefore the dominant factors determining the choice to computerize among New Jersey healthcare sectors.

Focus Group Results

Focus groups present excellent opportunities to elicit contextual nuances difficult to extract from factual surveys. Thus, eight focus groups were conducted to tap providers, payers, employers and public policy influencers views about EDI's potential in healthcare administrative functions. In the initial discussion phase, the focus group leader needed to establish the level of computer knowledge of the participants in each focus group. This initial discussion showed that computers were well known to nearly all participants as they use both paper and electronic media to accomplish their administrative tasks. Computer to computer interactive systems are very rare however. Most participants who exchange data with other organisations use tapes or disks. This is the same response found in the mail survey. Several findings from the focus groups are particularly relevant to this discussion of obstacles to EDI. Participants recognise that electronic systems are moving into all aspects of healthcare. They perceive a variety of obstacles to EDI, notably concerns about the complexity of the technology, fears that jobs will be lost, and recognition that people are slow to adapt to new ways. Smaller providers express concern about the costs associated with conversion from paper systems to electronic. Furthermore, they are faced with a wide variety of options that are expensive and require them to choose among proprietary technologies. They are unsure of the direction of future technology and fear that if they select a technology now, its early obsolescence will require additional costs to adapt to a new technology. The fear of additional expense also causes resistance among larger providers, who fear that EDI technology will require expensive hardware and software additions to existing technology.

In summary, the focus groups revealed that knowledge of computers and the technology of computer to computer communication is reasonably well spread within New Jersey's healthcare industry. And, many industry participants recognise and show concern for the threats it poses for their organisations. Since no standards exist, the existing plethora of proprietary technologies is causing providers to postpone further computerisation. On another level, they expect employee resistance to further computer technology changes at least partly because of the concern for job security. In other words, these providers, payers and business/government leaders have three fears about the adoption of EDI. Fear that their costs will increase. Fear that new technologies will create employee resistance to change and present the same problems that past and present proprietary technologies have given them. Fear that whatever technology they adopt will become obsolete and they will have to change again.

Conclusions About Obstacles

WEDI's comprehensive list makes it clear that there are technical reasons why EDI has not emerged naturally in the healthcare industry. WEDI's list differs from New Jersey's list in that WEDI's survey was largely conducted among technology experts whereas New Jersey's focus groups were with providers, payers and public policy decision makers. The New Jersey focus groups show that there are major concerns with costs and resistance of their organisations to the introduction of yet another technology to be followed too quickly by yet another. These fears are preventing many from moving forward with advanced computerisation and when coupled with the lack of technological standards, are simply making EDI an unacceptable technology. Obviously, like the WEDI survey respondents, New Jersey healthcare participants do not perceive appropriate incentives to adopt EDI. Without adequate assurances of well-defined, guaranteed, non-proprietary, technology standards and clear evidence of cost savings associated with such technology, New Jersey providers and payers have no meaningful incentives to overcome their fears and adopt EDI.

Discussion

The summary conclusion that can be drawn from the analysis in this chapter, based on material in previous and subsequent chapters, is that the major barrier to EDI adoption in the healthcare industry is the absence of appropriate incentives at the individual organisation level to accomplish the social goal of system-wide administrative cost reductions that EDI offers. The absence of incentives is expressed nationally as a combination of technical and human factors and among New Jersey healthcare industry participants as three fears related to their experiences: fear of costs; fear of new technologies; and fear of technology's early obsolescence. For some providers, the first two fears, of costs and of technology, are related. Their view of the costs of technology incorporates their recognition that the use of new technology requires considerable retraining. Thus, to them costs of adoption of technological solutions combines both the price of hardware and software (which has been declining) and the time and energy required to learn the technology. This latter is a growing factor as computer technologies become more sophisticated. The third fear, that of technological obsolescence, compounds the first two.

Most providers, especially those in larger organisations, such as hospitals, physician group practices, and payers, have ample experience with computer technologies. They have seen the rapid pace of technological change make yesterday's expensive decision to adopt promising proprietary technology become today's' millstone as the technology becomes obsolete. So, the wise and weary wait. Many of these same providers know how the promised cost savings of new technology can disappear in the training and re-training of personnel to accommodate a new computer system. Or they recognise that legal constraints make it too risky to initiate a cooperative effort within or across sectors. For other providers, the fear of costs is combined with the recognition that today's technology choice may be rendered obsolete by subsequent political decisions. So they wait also. Sociologists call these human barriers "resistance to change." But this is not the resistance of inexperienced or ignorant administrators. This is resistance built upon substantial knowledge and practical experience. These are economically prudent decisions of managers optimizing their organisation's individual position. Economically independent, prudent providers who optimize also inadvertently progress toward a technologically attainable legitimate social goal, i.e., reduction of administrative costs in the healthcare industry through adoption of EDI.

It also is obvious that the historical process of separate, independent, individual decisions will not eliminate these barriers, at least not in the foreseeable future. What individual decision makers in this fragmented industry need is a situation wherein technological development is defined such that their investments in technology will be reasonable, financially attractive and long-lived. This means proprietary systems must not dominate the technology. Instead, standardized systems with open, published procedures for connecting and using the systems are required. Furthermore, new technology must be adaptable to existing technology so additional costs are minimized. Costs of adopting the technology, especially training costs, must be reasonable. And, last but perhaps most important, documentable cost savings must be available to the individual user. These requirements for adopting new technologies have not yet been met by EDI proponents. Here the existing fragmented structure of the healthcare industry, so liked by American consumers and so much a part of American culture, has failed to identify an economically attractive mechanism to rise to the challenge. Thus, it is not surprising that the healthcare industry has not adopted EDI. Furthermore, without economic incentives to overcome the fears that dominate their decisions, America's independent entity system may collapse under the weight of rising demands for information to which it inefficiently responds. Then proponents of vertical integration may succeed in advocating hierarchical responses.

CURRENT STATE OF INFORMATION TECHNOLOGY

Technological advances in the prevention and treatment of trauma and disease in the last fifty years have significantly increased both the life span and the quality of life. Some of these advances are directly related to the availability of computers to collect, analyse and display data in a timely and cost effective manner. However, the technology that enables researchers to model the reaction of human cells to anti-bodies and view the interior of the body with Magnetic Resonance Imaging (MRI) has not been effectively applied to collection and storage of clinical records nor to the transmission of clinical and business information between health service providers, purchasers, and payers. As described in previous chapters, two closely linked, major factors have impeded information storage and data flow in the medical community:

1. Lack of standards for collection, storage, and transmission of data.
2. Competitiveness among the multiple participants in the healthcare industry.

This is not to say that computers are not widely used in the healthcare industry. As noted in this study, in New Jersey, 86 percent of hospitals, 33 percent of physicians, 40 percent of laboratories, and 89 percent of pharmacies are computerized. Still, with the exception of pharmacies, the vast majority of this computerisation is proprietary in nature and have limited ability for inter-computer communication. In other words, few physician computers can communicate directly with hospital computers. Nor can the physician computers communicate with pharmacies. This lack of inter-computer communication is particularly annoying in the healthcare industry because it is a fragmented industry made up of many separate business entities that are highly dependent upon each other to deliver services to their mutual patients. Few industries in the U.S. experience the high degree of fragmentation. So the healthcare industry, more than any other, needs inter-entity computerized communication, i.e., electronic data interchange (EDI). EDI offers the potential for linking the independent entities in the industry into a cost saving computer to computer communications network. Experience demonstrates that adequate computer technology currently exists to implement EDI. In fact, application of this technology to computerized communications of healthcare data already exists in New Jersey. For example, Blue Cross/Blue Shield of New Jersey has had computer terminals in most major New Jersey hospitals for many years. These terminals allow hospital personnel to electronically update Blue Cross claims that were submitted directly on computer tapes without paper. Another example, noted in study, is NEIC Incorporated, a Secaucus, New Jersey "claims clearinghouse," jointly owned by five healthcare payers. NEIC transmits claims electronically from its computers to the payers' computers. It provides this claims transmission service for healthcare provider organisations in nine states. NEIC receives paper or electronic claims information from providers. NEIC clerks convert the paper into electronic claims format. Then, NEIC's computers reformat the electronic claims to each payer's specific claim format and forward the electronic claims to the payers using each payer's computer specific communication protocol, i.e., the pattern of characters that define the data.

Similar Blue Cross services and NEIC like clearinghouses exist around the country. Providers willingly pay for Blue

Cross terminals and claims clearinghouse operators to perform this service because claims submission is so specialized that it is too expensive and complex for providers to do themselves. This cost and complexity is caused by the plethora of differing formats of claim forms required by the payers. Cook reports that there are 450 different claim forms required by some 3000 payers in the U.S. [1993, p. 3]. But, even the clearinghouses offer only a small percentage of the 450 claim forms. Providers must be prepared to file some claims by hand regardless of the number of clearing houses to which they subscribe.

Neither Blue Cross nor clearinghouses are true EDI operations because human intervention is still required in a significant share of the providers' claims processing activities. Blue Cross terminals do not accept initial claims submissions from providers, only changes to claims previously submitted. And, although clearinghouses process claims for numerous payers, clerks are still required to take paper submitted data and reformat it into proprietary formats and data transmission protocols to accommodate different (and competitive) payer organisations. since clearinghouses do not provide claims service for all payers, providers find they must subscribe to several clearinghouses and even then they are still required to have an in-house claims processing department that files paper claims with an additional set of payers. If a single *standardized claim form* existed and was uniformly accepted by all payers, along with a single *standardized data transmission protocol*, providers could easily train their own workers and programme their computer communications software to file claims electronically. Obviously, *standards* are the key to EDI. Standard forms and standard transmission protocols define EDI because EDI does not require new or special design hardware, communications networks nor unusual software.

All the necessary hardware is currently available from numerous suppliers. Communication networks currently exist. No unusual software is required. EDI will emerge as soon as standards are defined. When EDI is in place, providers and payers will experience considerable savings in administrative costs. Without standardized formats for transactions and protocols for transmissions, EDI cannot exist and healthcare administrative costs will remain high.

The purpose of this chapter is to describe and explain the current condition of computer technologies available for application to the healthcare industry in New Jersey and how these technologies can be developed into EDI through the adoption of standards. We begin with a description of computer communication technologies and their existence in various healthcare segments today. We examine the emerging standards for computerized data collection, storage and transmission that define future directions for computer use in the healthcare industry. We will show that administrative data collection, storage and transmission standards are currently well advanced as described in this study. Clinical data standards are not as well developed as we will demonstrate in this chapter. Other standards ancillary to EDI are also being developed and are discussed. We take up the issue of patient cards and their applications in the healthcare industry. Card based computer technologies have achieved an advanced degree of standardisation as evident by the wide spread use of uniformly designed bank and credit cards by millions of consumers. It seems natural to assume that such cards can be useful and offer cost reduction advantages in the healthcare industry just as they have brought reduced costs and greater convenience to consumer finance transactions. All of these technologies need to be examined for their influence on the question of patient information security.

We examine the computer security systems that are available to prevent unauthorized access to and use of computerized patient data. We examine the alternate views concerning individual privacy and the use of the Social Security Account Number as a common healthcare identifying number. We provide an example of a healthcare transaction system that can be implemented with currently available technologies. This is provided to demonstrate that existing technologies will support a fully integrated electronic data interchange system that will significantly reduce administrative costs in New Jersey.

Computer Communications

As evident in its name, EDI (electronic data interchange) involves the transmission of data between separate computers. Transmission is an act of communication. Thus, computer communication technologies are an over-riding consideration in evaluating current technologies available for EDI in health care. To explore this subject.

Electronic Networks

What is an electronic network? The phrase has many different definitions in the world of automation, and its meaning has changed as technology has developed. Initially, computing was only done on large mainframe computers that, due to their expense and the specialized environments required for their operation, were centralized. During this period, electronic networks referred to the system of terminals that were connected to a central mainframe computer and distributed in a variety of locations. The single purpose of the network was to link terminals to a host computer that provided a particular service or a set of services. As computer technologies became more developed, computer capacity increased while costs came down. With lower costs, more machines appeared and more applications were developed. As these developments took place, a change occurred in the use of networks. Powerful but inexpensive microcomputers could not only communicate with mainframes and each other, but could move data to and from other computers and process this data on these desktop machines. They could also provide many other capabilities which heretofore only mainframes could do. With these developments, multiple computers, instead of mainframes, became the central part of electronic networks. Initially, the quantity of data being transferred was small and data transfer rates (data per unit of time) were low but satisfactory for small data volumes. But as applications requiring large data transfer became popular, interest shifted to increasing the data transfer rate of the devices. Thus evolved, the megabits per second and gigabits per second networks. As these data transfer rates became available, users began to transfer even more data and electronic networks blossomed into international linkages. These linkages operate without a single central computer but instead use an electronic network of machines, each supporting itself and all others in the network. This basically describes the evolution of computer networks, an evolution that continues.

Types of Networks

To simplify the discussion we will categorize networks into four types: terminal, local area, wide area, and national/global.

Terminal Networks: Initially a terminal was directly connected to a computer. With the advent of more sophisticated computers, more than one terminal could be connected to a machine at one time using 'time sharing'. Time sharing means that each terminal user 'shared' a portion of the computing time of the computer. The physical range of these early networks was limited to about 250 feet and each terminal required a direct connection to the computer. Repeaters and concentrators were added to increase the distance and allow more than one terminal to share a line over the increased distance. Modems were subsequently invented so that telephone lines could be used to connect remotely located terminals to central computers. Modems are devices that convert the electronic signals produced by pressing the terminal keys into a series of pulses that can be transmitted on a telephone line. The modem also converts received pulses into characters displayed on the terminal screen. With a modem on a distant terminal and another on the computer, terminals could talk to computers over great distances on conventional telephone lines. Other computer type machines were invented to extend the distance and allow multiple users to share the same telephone line. However, all terminals were still connected to a single computer.

Local Area Networks (LANs): The development of Ethernet by Xerox and Digital Equipment Corporation enabled multiple devices to share a common wire, in this case a coaxial cable. A driving force behind Ethernet LANs was the development of the Computer Aided Design workstation, a very powerful microcomputer specialized for engineering design work. Each workstation had a unique digital "address," thereby enabling one workstation to send data to any other on the network without involving or passing through any other computer. This allowed the development of a whole new concept of a network. No longer was it necessary to have a central processor to identify and route communications from one terminal to another. Each workstation could route its own communications. Thus, a central computer was no longer required for routing. However, it was useful to have file servers, print servers and eventually E-mail servers. "Servers" are separate computers that serve to store files for workstation users to access, receive print commands and schedule these into one or more printers, and to receive and store electronic messages from one workstation to another if the receiving workstation is busy. In addition, terminal servers were developed which enable `dumb' terminals (or workstations that want to perform as dumb terminals) to use the same cable to communicate with mainframes and minicomputers. Subsequently, networks were adopted by business organisations using PCs and Macintosh machines. Today, PCs, Macintoshes and workstations can communicate directly with each other and establish cooperative computing environments such as client-server architectures with little problem. In a client-server network architecture, the data entry, editing and display are managed at the individual computer (client) while the server controls common functions (e.g., printing, E-mail, etc.) and databases for all clients. A local area network can span 1000 feet or more allowing an entire floor or small building to be serviced by one LAN. The speed is usually 10 Megabits per second (10 Mbs) for Ethernet and 4 or 16 Mbs per second for Token Ring. Hardware (repeaters) currently exists to boost the distance over which LANs can communicate. It seems appropriate here to digress into the subject of communication protocols. Networks cannot work without standard definitions of the type of data bits traveling down the wire. The standard definitions are important and are discussed next.

Network Protocols: The exchange of data between network connected computers is controlled by a set of rules, a network protocol that specifies how messages are prepared and transmitted electronically. A computer programme might want to transfer to another computer a simple communication such as a patient's medical record number, but the actual exchange of data consists solely of electrical signals. The nature of these electronic signals must be defined in advance with the receiving computer so that the signals can be "read" by the receiving computer as a patient medical record number. This "electronic signal definition" is called a communication protocol. The International Standards Organisation (ISO) has developed a communications model, Open Systems Interconnect (OSI), that organises the protocols involved in transforming the data constructs into electrical signals. The protocol rules are organised into seven layers. At the lowest levels, protocols define the physical connections, the packet formats, the means of addressing packets, and the timing and sequencing of transmission. Each layer services the layer above it and expects certain functions or services from the layer below it. Data exchange standards being developed for healthcare deal primarily with OSI Layers 7 and 6 (Application and Presentation). The OSI model defines an application process as "an element within an open system which performs the information processing for a particular application" [Stallings, 1990]. The application processes themselves lie outside the seven-layer OSI architecture. Applications include claims transmission, eligibility inquiries, electronic payment transfers, etc. The *OSI application layer* provides services to these application processes and provides the means for application processes to access the OSI environment. The application layer service elements can be thought of as providing useful services that are relevant to one or more application processes.

The purpose of the *OSI presentation layer* is to assure that end systems may successfully communicate even if they use different representations. It does this by providing a common representation to be used in communication and by converting from the local representation to this common representation. The syntax used between two presentation entities is referred to as the transfer syntax. This is the common representation. The OSI model does not specify a single predetermined transfer syntax. Instead the syntax used on a particular presentation connection is negotiated dynamically between the two communicating systems. At the application layer, information is represented in an abstract syntax that deals with data types and data values. An abstract syntax has many similarities to the data type definitions of common programming languages. The presentation layer translates between the abstract syntax of the application layer and a transfer syntax that describes the data values in a binary form which is then passed on to the next lower OSI level, the session level. Encoding rules are used to transform the abstract syntax to the transfer syntax. Although the OSI model has been in existence since 1978, there are few implementations that make use of all seven layers. There are other de facto standards, such as, IBM's Systems Network Architecture (SNA) and Transmission Control Protocol/Internet Protocol (TCP/IP) that are well entrenched and will probably persist if not flourish. Most OSI implementations have made use of certain OSI layers on top of SNA or TCP/IP. For example, Marshall Rose has the ISO Development Environment, which consists of fully compliant OSI application and presentation layers that operate on top of TCP/IP services [Rose, 1990]. The OSI model has also been used extensively as a way of describing existing systems that are not themselves OSI compliant. One way or another, all networked computing systems perform the functions outlined in the OSI model, but they might not be structured as a seven layer system. In such systems, the functions of several layers might be so tightly coupled that they can not be separated out. In a truly OSI compliant system each layer can be exchanged for another piece of software that performs the same function and none of the other layers would be aware of the change. This is the principle proposed benefit to systems that implement the OSI model.

Now an example, in this case, sending a message that states a patient's current location in a hospital or clinic. In the ideal case, the two communicating applications (terminals or PCs) should behave as if they were directly transferring data between themselves. They should not be concerned with the transformation of the information as it is packaged in a form that can traverse the network. These services are performed by the lower six layers. In this scenario, developing standards for the exchange of healthcare data would consist solely of specifying the actual information that has to be transferred between applications. For example, to send a patient's current location, the applications would only have to settle on a standard representation for a patient identification number and a way of representing locations. This information might be combined in some sort of message that the two applications would send to each other. All other formatting issues would be dealt with by the standards for the lower layers. Therefore, application developers could concentrate their efforts on developing specific application level protocol standards.

Now, back to networks.

Wide Area Networks (WANs): A Wide Area Network (WAN) is often simply a series of LANs connected to a common "backbone". The backbone is the linkage among the LANs and may, or may not, have some devices directly attached to it. The backbone may in fact be nothing more than communication lines leased from a public service carrier (e.g., telephone company). The backbone may be several parallel or interconnecting lines using copper wires, coax cable, glass fiber cable, microwave transmitters/receivers, or satellite transmission. In any case, the user company is the manger of the network and the carrier is simply a service provider. As with LANs, if the WAN has a variety of computer hardware connected to it, it will have the appropriate hardware and have a standard six layers communication protocol established so all hardware connected to the WAN can communicate with all other connected hardware. One of the early problems for WAN developers was interconnecting different types of LANs. LANs which utilize different protocols cannot routinely exchange data because the electronic characteristics and even the stream of data bits used on one LAN are not understood by the other LAN. This problem was solved by installing "routers" between the LANs. Routers are translators that receive electrical signals (and now also light pulses over fiber optic cables) and convert the signals into data bits that can be forwarded to the other LAN. Most routers can connect multiple LANs simultaneously enabling computers to send messages to any computer on any other connected LAN without the need to develop individual connection hardware or software. Routers serve two additional functions: segmenting and providing a "firewall".

Segmenting is the dividing of a WAN or even a large LAN into smaller segments to reduce the communications traffic on the individual segments and thereby increase the efficiency of the WAN or LAN. By segmenting, only the traffic for an individual segment is carried on that segment. Only messages addressed from a computer on one segment to a computer on another segment pass through the router. The term 'firewall' is copied from the construction term meaning 'a partition between two adjacent parts of a building that inhibits the spread of fire from one section to the other. The computer firewall is a device that keeps unauthorized computers (individuals) from using a computer, observing the traffic or determining the configuration of the network within the boundary protected by the firewall. A router is a starting point for a fire wall. A firewall greatly enhances the security with the protected boundary. The inherent design of routers, i.e. segregation of traffic, when coupled with security software, can provide the protection called a firewall. A router used as a firewall will only pass traffic in and out of the protected segment through one point. The computer receiving traffic from the outside also performs firewall functions by insuring that the traffic originates with a legitimate user and carries no hidden virus.

National / Global Networks: The Advanced Research Projects Agency Network (ARPANet) which is the foundation for the Internet is the most widely recognised network in the U.S. The Internet is an interconnection of multiple network providers who allow users to connect to an individual network and send and receive data to any point on any part of the network. The major difference between a WAN and the Internet is that the individual networks that comprise the Internet are organisations from whom LAN, and WAN users buy services. The communication protocol is standardized for the Internet.

National Research and Education Network (NREN) is a first step in the process of building a national data highway [Wrubel, 1993]. It is a federally funded gigabit-speed networking programme. Some refer to NREN as a national information super highway. NREN will eventually be a gigabit network that will transmit a billion bits of information or more per second. The thought of NREN as a national information infrastructure is very exciting but most of it's details are yet to be specified. Initially, the major goal of NREN is to create a high-speed computing network among dozens of government labs, agencies and institutions such as the Department of Energy, the Department of Defense and the National Aeronautics and Space Administration [Wrubel, 1993]. However, ultimately research labs, universities, libraries, hospitals, businesses and eventually consumers will be connected into this vast high speed computing network capable of shipping billions of bits of digital information anywhere in the country on fiber optic cables. According to the National Science Foundation (NSF), NREN will evolve out of a network currently referred to as Interagency Interim NREN (otherwise known as NSFNet). This NSF network, operating on the Internet T3 backbone at 45 Mbs, spans the country and NSF is planning to boost it's data rate to 155 Mbs over a next few years [Lloyd, 1992]. NREN is already a commercially viable information highway if one accepts the NSFNet portion of the Internet as the core of NREN. NREN today consists of the NSFNet backbone and five gigabit test beds. By 1996, the NSFNet will run at 155 Mbs or faster and will be joined with the test-beds which will be operating at 1.2 Gigabits per second or higher [Ahiswede, et.al., 1993].

Networks for Health Care

Current networks for healthcare range from terminal networks connected to a single mainframe, to a LAN for group medical practice, to WANs for large teaching hospitals. For example, the Blue Cross claims filing network is a terminal network. LANs are common in group practices where two or more PCs work together on a practice management system. Recently, WAN type interconnections between providers and payers have been established in the NEIC clearinghouse network described earlier. However, the NEIC network acts as a central point clearing house for proprietary transactions and does not provide the end-to-end communications of an EDI system.

Paper versus Electronic Networks: Transport of healthcare information, on computer networks can save millions of dollars yearly. As stated by Kadas and Butler the growing burden of data on claims is as follows:

> Patients and healthcare providers file billions of insurance claims annually. Industry experts estimate that electronic filing (with use of computer networks) could cut costs by as much as $2 per claim, saving about $8 billion in national healthcare costs annually, according to the Health Insurance Association of America.

Large numbers of electronic claim formats are now in use by payers throughout the nation, but it is still not sufficient.

- — Most private claims submitted manually take, on average, between 12 to 25 days to process. Electronic filing cuts processing time to about 10 days and is considerably more accurate.
- — Health and Human Services officials note that by incorporating electronic funds transfer services into a nationwide electronic claims system, administrative costs of paying claims will drop from a current average of 29 cents per transaction to just 3 to 10 cents. In addition, providers will have quicker access to their money and be assured funds are deposited. The Health Care Financing Administration wants to implement direct deposit as soon as possible.

The Health Care Finance Administration (HCFA), the federal agency that manages the financial aspects of Medicare, has created a strategic plan to increase electronic claims. According to HCFA, the agency now receives more than 75 percent of all hospital and 44 percent of other claims electronically. This indicates that people do realise the importance of transferring healthcare information data on networks and much work has been done in this direction [Kadas and Butler, 1992].

Medical Network Characteristics: What should be the characteristics of a medical communication network: According to Hanlon and Kaskiw [1992]:

The network should be designed to enhance the efficiency and effectiveness of communication among the hospitals, specialists and primary-care physician. Its main application should be interconnecting hospitals and physicians over normal dial-up telephone lines. It could be used to deliver automatic lab and radiology reports, patient information, referral and admission information, selected clinical graphics and digitized voice file. In addition to these, medical communication networks should be capable of shipping images such as x-rays and MRIs and also have the capability to carry video conferencing so specialists could meet and discuss a case without traveling to a single location. Such a network should be *open* to all legitimate users. Open means that any computer programmed with the network protocol will have access to the network. This is the way the Internet works today. This is also true of the Prodigy, American On-line, and Delphi networks. Anyone who acquires the network protocol software, identifies the connection point, and pays the fee can connect and use the network. Such an advanced health information network could be used to send data from physicians' offices to hospitals or vice versa. A physician can use the system to schedule referral appointments for his patients with specialists, send patient records and test results to other physicians and receive test results as soon as they are transcribed. Paper reports that take weeks to reach their destination can arrive in minutes [Marcotta, 1989]. The hospital-physician computer link is one of the most popular applications in the healthcare industry. Such communications can reduce physician time and improve patient care because of the immediacy of information availability. Physicians like the time saving aspects of such communications while hospitals see hospital based systems as cementing relations between specialists, primary-care physicians and hospitals [Gardner and Perry, 1990].

Advantages of NREN for a National Healthcare System: Currently, the Internet, but eventually NREN, provide an appropriate network for the healthcare industry's EDI needs. Perhaps separate WANs or LANs will also be used locally but a fully operational EDI system will require a national network like Internet or NREN. The advantages of an EDI system operating on NREN will be the *open* nature of the system. Eventually, all the many participants in the fractured healthcare industry will be connected to the network. Like all networks, all messages carry an address that directs the message to the specific computer for which it is intended. To send a message, a computer merely needs to know the correct address. And all computers are continuously connected so all messages are delivered immediately. For example, a physician's computer can send a claim to one payer, make a eligibility inquiry to another payer, receive a lab report from a pathologist, and receive a patient referral from another physician all within seconds, all from the same network connection, all automatically. No human is needed to answer the "phone", make notes or confirm the validity of the information. All transactions are verified by the computers involved.

Image transmission such as X-rays, MRIs, and even magnifications of cell sections require much greater transmission capacity than is available on Internet. However, NREN will have more than enough capacity as identified in test carried out in NJIT's lab. Such EDI technology can be used to solve problems of high costs and inadequate access currently dogging the national healthcare system. A study conducted by the consulting firm Arthur D. Little Inc.,

Cambridge, MA, supports this view. The study projects that U.S. healthcare costs could be trimmed by more than $36 billion annually through wide spread electronic management of patient information, electronic claims processing, electronic inventory procedures and video conferencing. Little's predictions of annual savings through wider use of telecommunications is as follows [Little, 1992].

- — $30 billion Electronic management of patient information
- — $6 billion Electronic claims processing
- — $0.6 billion Electronic inventory controls
- — $0.2 billion Video conferencing

Savings are also projected to result from early intervention in medical problems, fewer patient visits to emergency departments and clinics and directing patients to the most appropriate level of care. Improving the flow of information between hospitals and physicians is especially critical for these savings to be realised.

Electronic Data Interchange

EDI is the electronic exchange of business information in a standard format. In the healthcare industry, "business information" can include a variety of business data such as financial data, claims, benefit inquiries, payment receipts and payments made, purchase orders, and invoices. However, it may also include administrative data such as enrollment information, eligibility verification, provider referrals, and provider scheduling. In addition, healthcare EDI will eventually handle clinical data, such as prescriptions, medical tests, and medical records.

Although it relies on a combination of computer hardware, software and communication links with electronic document standards, rules and procedures, EDI is not, in itself, a computer system. EDI is a powerful business concept for utilizing today's electronic environment to automate and re-engineer business processes for maximum productivity and control. The concept of EDI is to standardize and automate business communications between all trading partners in a market sector through consensus on using a common "architecture" for electronic communication. As such, it provides the basis for industry to move from labor intensive, paper-based business processes into an automated system of electronic commerce. The architecture of EDI (standard document formats, standard network protocols, and open communications systems) can be applied effectively in electronic medical claims, purchasing and banking to improve present systems. Procedures such as eligibility inquiry and response, claims filing and payment advice, purchase orders, shipping notices, sales/price catalogues, invoices and payments can be automated with all trading partners using the same EDI "system", thus reducing costs and improving information flow. Implementing or converting to EDI does not require replacing existing computer application systems or extensive reprogramming. Rather, it uses

— a set of publicly known standards,
— agreements between trading partners on rules of exchange and business procedures,
— the enabling technology of EDI translation/ communications software, communication links, and
— EDI Value-Added Networks.

Standard electronic document formats are developed and published by the American National Standards Institute EDI Committee (known as ASC X12). Rules of exchange are outlined in published EDI document usage conventions. Business procedures are outlined in EDI Trading Partner Agreements. Commercially available EDI translation software enables the exchange of information with all other trading partners' applications (using standard public protocols) and eliminates the need of extensive reprogramming and support of application systems. EDI communications are set up via telephone lines between two firms and through Value-Added-Networks (VANs). VANs are used to solve interface and communication problems between multiple firms that have different computer systems, different protocols, and different schedules.

When a wide variety of organisations are involved in EDI, an open network is desirable with public communication protocols. This means that any computer can buy a connection and then transmit and receive on the network using the proper protocols and the standard data formats. This open system network is the obvious form for EDI in the healthcare industry. To accomplish this, standards are necessary for data and communication protocols.

Data Standards for Health Care

As noted above, the EDI communication of clinical and administrative data depends on the development of standards necessary to define the data formats and communication protocols. Presently, there is no master plan for such development. and no agreement among the many heterogeneous entities in the healthcare industry regarding EDI standards. So while proprietary LANs and WANs are operating in the healthcare industry today, standards for connecting these into open statewide, or even nationwide, networks do not exist. As noted in previous chapters, The Hartford Foundation, a not-for-profit foundation with interests in improving healthcare in America, recognised this problem four years ago. It has helped organise and fund several state projects designed to establish and implement EDI standards and networks. The Hartford Foundation calls these projects under their sponsorship Community Health Information Management Systems

(CHMIS). A CHMIS is an open EDI system with the short term focus of communicating administrative information and a long term focus of accumulating transmitted information in a data base for community health evaluation [Benton, 1992].

Interestingly, the Hartford Foundation early on accepted as reality the assumption that clinical data standards were becoming available far more slowly than administrative data standards. The Hartford Foundation recognised that there are far more problems with clinical data. For example, the current data storage systems for medical records are almost entirely paper and/or image (e.g., microfiche) type systems. Doctors' and nurses' hand written notes are common components. Printed computer reports are also common parts of a medical record. The printed computer reports appear because the computer systems that currently generate clinical data such as pathology test results, radiology X-rays and evaluations, cardiology analyses, pharmacy, etc., all operate with proprietary hardware/software that uses incompatible protocols so that electronic exchange of information is not possible. Thus, computer outputs are typically printed by the computer and stored on paper. X-rays and MRIs are printed and stored as sheets of film. All of this paper then becomes part of the medical record. Converting these images to computer readable form is complex and prone to significant errors. Thus, computerizing the medical record requires substantial changes in a multitude of clinical procedures that create the mass of paper. The standard setting process is extremely complex as we will show below. Administrative data, on the other hand, consists of some relatively common procedures shared by most providers and payers. Therefore, it is useful to explore in some detail the difference between administrative and clinical data standards in order to project the eventual availability of such standards and the probable timing of their arrival in network usable form. This section begins with a description of the overall effort to develop computing/communicating standards in the healthcare industry. This section concludes with a descriptive list of all the standards setting organisations that are involved.

The Need for Data Standards

Useful EDI provides data exchange in a way that is transparent to the user. The telephone system is a good example of system transparency. Massive telephone networks of computers, cables and switches lie behind every telephone call, but the user simply dials a number and hears a voice. No evidence of the complex technology is apparent during the conversation. The phone call appears to be a simple, uncomplicated process to the user. While it is true that there are innumerable standards for computer networks, much effort has been expended on developing systems and protocols that permit transparent communication between disparate systems. A prime example is the protocol referred to as TCP/IP (Transmission Control Protocol / Internet Protocol) [Comer, 1991]. This protocol is rapidly becoming a de facto standard for network communication and has been embraced by the majority of hardware vendors. However, the development of standards for the format and content of the data being communicated has lagged. What this means is that the computers can communicate, but application programmes—the stuff that users really want to see communicated—do not readily understand the data being transferred. So users find themselves working with the underlying technologies rather than transparently communicating. Development of application programmes that provide transparent user information communication suffer from two problems: inadequate data format standards and lack of vocabulary standards.

Data Format Standards

Standards are needed for both the format of the data being communicated and also for the vocabulary that is used to define medical knowledge such as tests, diagnoses, observations, medications, etc. The data format standard can be thought of as equivalent to the syntactical grammar of a language. When you read an English language sentence, you can identify the subject, verb and object, as well as other components of the sentence. This is the purpose of a data format standard. The data that flows between the communicating systems can be dissected into its component parts. For example, in a message that contains the name and current location of a patient, the receiving system should be able to easily extract the patient's name and location. The data format standard must also define a common representation for data, such as patient name, patient address, date and time, etc. There should be no ambiguities. Both sender and receiver are free to store the shared data in whatever form they so choose, but there is only one approved form that is shared and used for communication. For example, system A might store dates as DDMMYY and system B as MMDDYYYY, therefore, they cannot communicate date data unless they adopt a standard format (e.g., the ISO standard date format YYYYMMDD). Common data types that are already addressed by standards include: person name, address, sex, phone number, date, time, numeric, text, etc.

Vocabulary

The other part of data standards is the meaning of the character stream that appears in the defined field. The business vocabulary of name, address, phone, and sex, etc., are well defined by conventional use. On the other hand, the vocabulary of medicine is not so well defined. Suppose that two systems are attempting to transfer a list of diagnoses for a given patient. System A has stored the patient's diagnoses as a list of International Classification of Disease (ICD-9-CM) codes, but System B has no knowledge of ICD-9-CM and stores its diagnoses in the format known as Systematized Nomenclature for Human and Veterinary Medicine (SNOMED) codes. While the two systems could communicate the list of diagnoses via a common data format standard, System B has no means of understanding or processing ICD-9-CM codes, i.e., vocabulary. While a standard for codes and vocabularies would greatly facilitate transparent data exchange, there has yet to emerge a single encompassing medical vocabulary standard. Currently, there are numerous vocabularies and nomenclatures for expressing medical information so most applications developers have to build translation tables that map one vocabulary to another. Viewing this as a significant problem in healthcare computing, the National Library of Medicine (NLM) has undertaken the development of the Unified Medical Language System (UMLS) [Humphreys and Lindberg, 1989]. This is not an attempt to impose a standard vocabulary, but it represents an effort to deal effectively with the continued diversity in medical terminology by creating a thesaurus of terms. The primary objective of the Metathesaurus of the UMLS is to permit cross referencing (mapping in computer terminology) between the many different sets of terminology, i.e., MeSH, DSM-IIIR, COSTAR, ICD-9-CM, SNOMED, CPT-4 and LCSH terms. However, there are still some in the field who believe that for computerisation of the patient medical record to become a reality there needs to be a single standard vocabulary for expressing medical information. No doubt the plethora of vocabularies listed above make it clear that the eventual adoption of a standard medical vocabulary is a long way away. As mentioned earlier, vocabulary is not a problem for administrative data, therefore, the remainder of this section will deal primarily with administrative data format standards which are further along the development path.

Coordination of the Standard Setting Efforts

There have been some attempts at coordinating the efforts of the various standards groups. Several of these, Health Level 7, American Society for Testing Materials (ASTM) and the IEEE Medical Data Interchange (MEDIX) Committee have numerous members in common and have formed convergence subcommittees in each group. Additionally, a joint committee called the healthcare Information Standards Coordinating Committee (HISCC) was formed in January, 1988 to provide a forum for the exchange of information regarding the development of standards for healthcare information systems [Harrington, et.al., 1989]. Much information has been shared and several actions toward convergence have occurred, but little real progress has been made. In October, 1990 the secretary general of the European Committee for Standardisation asked the American National Standards Institute to find a mechanism for providing a coordinated U.S. response to the European Committee for Standardisation's Technical Committee on medical informatics. This European group is very active and has seven working groups and a large number of project teams.

In March, 1991 a meeting was sponsored by the Agency for Health Care Policy and Research in cooperation with the American National Standards Institute (ANSI) and the Food and Drug Administration. Most of the standards groups and numerous government organisations sent representatives. ANSI recommended that a healthcare informatics planning panel be formed. The formation of a planning panel is a mechanism that ANSI uses to foster collaboration in a field when there are several groups developing overlapping standards. The vote was overwhelmingly in favour of forming the panel. A follow-up meeting was held in August 1991 at the ANSI headquarters in New York. The purpose of this meeting was to elicit a wider participation by other standards groups and to discuss the few negative votes. This time the vote was unanimous and the motion to create an ANSI Planning Panel was proposed to the ANSI Executive Committee. This was approved on January 22, 1992., and the formation of the Health Informatics Standards Planning Panel (HISPP) was announced by ANSI.

Health Informatics Standards Planning Panel (HISPP)

The planning panel was established to perform the function of a Standards Planning Panel per Section C2.3 of the ANSI Procedures for Development and Coordination of American National Standards (ANS) in the field of healthcare informatics. Specifically, the planning panel was to coordinate the work of the standards groups for healthcare data interchange and healthcare informatics and other relevant standards groups toward achieving the evolution of a unified set of non-redundant, non-conflicting standards that are compatible with ISO and non-ISO communications environments. In addition, a balanced subcommittee of the planning panel will interact with and provide input to the European Standards Committee in a coordinated fashion and explore avenues of international development [ANSI, 1991].

The standards with which HISPP is concerned are [ANSI, 1991]:

— Health care models and electronic healthcare records.
— The interchange of healthcare data, images, sounds and signals within and between organisations and practices.
— Health care codes and terminology.

— The communication with diagnostic instruments and healthcare devices.
— The representation and communication of healthcare protocols, knowledge, and statistical data bases.
— Privacy, confidentiality and security of medical information.
— Additional areas of concern and interest with regard to healthcare information.

The HISPP has meetings two to three time a year. Meetings have been attended by the voting members and other non-voting attendees (observers, liaisons to the HISPP and ANSI staff). Its members are classified into seven categories [ANSI, 1991]:

— Producers/manufacturers
— Standards developing organisations
— Professional societies
— Trade associations
— Government/regulatory agencies
— Users
— General interest

With regard to data exchange standards, the most important work of the Panel so far has been the formation of the ANSI healthcare Message Standards Developers Subcommittee (MSDS). The representatives of all of the standards groups have agreed to separate the information content from the interchange format, so that decisions about the interchange format can be made independently of the content standards. Some of the groups will convert their syntax to X12 [ANSI, 1992]. Some of the groups will not commit to X12 until a few questions are answered, but will work toward the use of a common syntax model. The groups have also agreed to divide up the message content into separate functional areas. The task of each group will be to define the data model specific to their functional area and specify the data elements within messages related to their functional areas. The groups also agreed to develop common logical representations for ubiquitous data elements such as persons, codes for defining procedures, tests, diagnoses, dates, etc., and a common set of codes for identifying source books for codes. Responsibilities have been divided up and given to the standards organisations that are a part of HISPP. First, Health Level 7 (HL7) has been assigned institution financial transactions, order entry, nursing management, automatic data transfer intra-institution, and appointment scheduling. Second, the American College of Radiologists jointly with the National Electrical Manufacturers Association (ACR-NEMA) are responsible for diagnostic images and communications within Picture Archiving and Communication Systems (PACS). Fourth, the American Society for Testing Materials (ASTM) is responsible for results of non-image clinical and nursing observations obtained by testing and diagnostic studies, or by providers such as nurses, respiratory therapists, physicians (including history and physical) [ANSI, 1992].

Fifth, the American National Standards Institute X12 committee (ANSI X12) is responsible for translating data content as it applies to intra-institutional communication into X12 syntax. It is also responsible for billing and insurance issues within an institution, physician and institutional billing information sent to third party payers, verification of coverage, and purchasing with all associated external documents. Sixth, the National Council for Prescription Drug Programmes (NCPDP) is responsible for intra-institutional pharmacy transactions. And seventh, the Institute of Electrical and Electronics Engineers (IEEE) Medical Data Interchange (MEDIX) Committee is responsible for acute care devices, all ISO and OSI related issues, including other interchange formats. IEEE will also coordinate the global data model [ANSI, 1992]. All those involved with this process so far are very optimistic that there is a good sound platform for future negotiations. The presence of the HISPP panel and its goal of "...achieving the evolution of a unified set of non-redundant, non-conflicting standards..." should be a clear sign to all those who are working toward that the healthcare informatics community is moving forward in a coordinated manner. The formation of the MSDS subcommittee and its progress are strong indicators that the process is working. In fact, the MSDS subcommittee has recently setup an anonymous file transfer protocol server for sharing documents, programmes and other material associated with standards for electronic data exchange. It will be through efforts like this that "...uniform national standards for data and security [will] facilitate implementation of the computerized patient record and its secondary databases" [Dick and Steen, 1991].

ANSI HISPP Subcommittees

The current HISPP efforts have been organised into two major subcommittees, the Message Standards Developers Subcommittee (MSDS) and the International and Regional Standards Issues (ISC) Subcommittee. The HISPP MSDS Subcommittee was formed in 1992 to coordinate and encourage cooperation and information exchange among the U.S. messaging standards developers. In order to examine message content from various functional areas, a network of joint working groups (JWGs) was established, each to work in a different functional area. The focus of each JWG was directed to one of the standards developing organisations charged with the task of defining the data model specific to their functional area and specifying the data elements within messages related to their functional area. These JWGs would also develop common logical representation for ubiquitous data elements such as persons, codes for defining procedures, test, diagnoses, dates, etc., and a common set of codes for identifying source books for codes. All developers participate in all JWGs and the results of each JWG is shared by all. Considerable progress has been made to date and a number of documents have been produced and circulated to HISPP [ANSI, 1992].

The HISPP International Standards Committee Subcommittee has been charged to interact with and provide input to the European Standards Committee in a coordinated fashion and to explore avenues of international standards development. This subcommittee is reviewing and determining U.S. positions on the European Standards and is exploring the formation of a possible ISO technical committee on this subject, discussing this possibility with experts in other countries to gain support for it. The HISPP and this subcommittee have reviewed a large number of documents of CEN TC-251 to date, and U.S. comments for submittal to the European Standards Committee have been developed on a number of these documents.

In the past two years, 1992 and 1993, in order to carry out its work HISPP has formed three task groups: [ANSI, 1993]

— The Codes and Vocabulary Task Group,
— The Privacy, Security and Confidentiality Task Group, and
— The Provider Identification Numbering Systems Task Group.

In addition, a special HISPP Task Group was recently formed, meeting for the first time on July 15, 1993, to address the U.S. government positions on Medical Informatics. A case in point is the report recently developed by the U.S. General Accounting Office for the U.S. Senate

Committee on Government Affairs, issued in April 1993, titled "Automated Medical Records - Leadership Needed to Expedite Standards Development" to which HISPP has prepared a response report stating its position. Not mentioned in the preceding review but emerging within the first half of 1994 is the role of WEDI as the standards setting sub-committee of ANSI X12. Thus, WEDI has become the healthcare administrative applications standard setting organisation thereby taking on a more important role than simply a watchdog for the administrative problems of the healthcare industry [WEDI, 1993].

Standards Development Techniques

At this point it may be useful to quickly review the basic OSI model of data communication layers. There are seven layers beginning (from the users perspective) with the application layer. Below the application layer are six more layers that must have standards established for EDI to take place. The application layer is where the user interfaces with the computer and where the computer performs the task the user desires. For example, if a nurse wishes to record the arrival of a patient within the boundaries of his/her responsibility, s/he accesses an application that carries out this function. To the nurse, communication is transparent. S/he enters the information on the local computer and assumes that it is received in a central record location. What the computer actually does is not important nor relevant to the nurse as long at the notification and recording process occurs as expected. Properly designed applications make the telecommunications transparent to the user.

Interestingly, the application layer is the most difficult to standardized because users have substantially different ways of doing their work. Furthermore, the reality of human behaviour in performing tasks is strikingly difficult for computers to perform. For example, in word processing, spell checking is a standard human function that is extremely difficult for computers. While a skilled human editor can glance across a paragraph and identify a misspelled word, the computer must examine every character of every word and match each word to its internal dictionary of all words to determine if the word is spelled correctly. Only the extremely high speed of modern computers (millions of instructions per second) makes spell checking appear to be rather human in its process. For this reason, many applications have been slow in developing into fully user friendly procedures that humans find useful. Application design is an important part of standards development. Applications developers have been forever plagued by the difficulty of building applications that truly function in a manner that is useful to the end-user. Not too infrequently, after an application has been running for a period of time, it is realised that the original design has a fundamental flaw that requires major modifications. The principal source of this problem is that it is very difficult to understand and model reality as perceived by a specially skilled end user. Computer application design tasks have long been done by computer experts, usually specialists in systems analysis and database administration, while reality exists in the work of end users such as professional medical workers and business managers. Historically, it was rare to find a mix of these computer system design skills and end user skills in the same person. Gradually, people with a mix of skills are becoming more common. The application design task has been deemed so difficult that it has been regarded more of an art than a science. Over the last two decades various methodologies have been developed to help in the modeling and design of applications. While it is true that most of these methodologies have been applied to database design, these methods can also be applied to other application design situations, including the design of data exchange standards. There will be no convergence of the current standards unless each group adopts formal design methodologies and together the groups arrive at a model for data exchange in the healthcare environment. The ultimate goal is that systems should be able to communicate healthcare data as easily as it is to purchase and plug together home electronic components. This has been termed "plug and play". The various groups have all realised that the adoption of formal design methodologies are required if this goal is to be realised. A design methodology is a structured approach for discovering, analysing, and modeling a set of requirements in a standardized, organised manner. A design methodology consists of several key ingredients. Of the eight ingredients listed below, the first six are mandatory, while the last two are optional [Fleming and von Halle, 1989]:

— Statement of objective
— Step-by-step procedure for establishing the objective
— Guidelines, or rules of thumb that accompany all transformation processes
— Standard and consistent documentation techniques
— Examples and an illustrative case study
— Assignment of roles and responsibilities for performing and reviewing each step
— Formal course instruction for transferring the methodology
— Computer-based tools to assign in the design process.

The current data exchange standards have suffered most from a lack of a comprehensive data model. Data models are vehicles for describing reality. Designers use data models to build schema's which are representations of reality. There are several methodologies for arriving at a data model. Currently in vogue are entity-relationship modeling and object-oriented analysis. While there are proponents of each method, the important thing will be that formal design methodologies are used to create data exchange standards and that the workers in this field abandon their current ad hoc methods [Batini, et.al., 1992]. Without a robust data model for communications in health care, EDI will remain elusive.

Standards Generating Organisations

As mentioned earlier, a number of committees and organisations are prominent in their work to develop healthcare informatics standards in the United States and thus their function falls under the HISPP coordination purview. These include:

- — American National Standards Accredited Standards Committee X3 (X3),
- — American National Standards Accredited Standards Committee X12 (X12),
- — American College of Radiology / National Electrical Manufacturers Association (ACR/NEMA),
- — ASTM Committee E31 (ASTM 31),
- — Health Level 7 (HL7),
- — Institute of Electrical and Electronics Engineers (IEEE),
- — Association For Information And Image Management (AIIM), and
- — National Council for Prescription Drug Programmes (NCPDP).

In the following paragraphs, these standards setting organisations will be described with emphasis upon their areas of specialisation and the standards that currently exist or are under development.

Accredited Standards Committee X3 (ASC X3 or just X3)

X3, administered by the Computer and Business

Equipment Manufacturers Association (CBEMA), is charged to develop generic standards for information technology, and is accredited to submit its documents to ANSI for approval as American National Standards. X3 has a very large work programme, and many of its documents are currently accepted as standards by American National Standards Institute. There is significant work under way which may be of specific interest to the healthcare informatics community. However, the X12 committee will incorporate the X3 standards as they become available so the X12 committee is far more important to EDI in health care.

Accredited Standards Committee X12 (ASC X12 or just X12)

X12 is administered by the Data Interchange Standards Association (DISA), and is accredited to submit its documents to ANSI for approval as American National Standards. X12 has written many standards specifications, e.g., for the banking industry, and many of its documents have been accepted by the American National Standards Institute. Of interest to the healthcare informatics community are the specifications and the documents being developed by the X12 Insurance Subcommittee on general healthcare communication standards but with a focus on insurance issues.

In particular ASC X12 has published the following standards:

— 835 Healthcare Claim Payment,
— 837 Healthcare Claim,
— 270 Eligibility Request,
— 271 Eligibility Response,
— 834 Enrollment,
— 148 Report of Injury or Illness,
— 186 Life and Annuity Lab Report.

ASC X12 is also working on the following:

— Coordination of Benefits,
— Claim Status Request and Response, and
— Patient Record Data Request and Response.

X12 is so important to the development of EDI within the healthcare industry that we devote an entire section to it later in this chapter.

American College of Radiologists / National Electrical Manufacturers Association (ACR/NEMA)

This is a joint effort between these two organisations to develop a standard for Digital Imaging and Communications in Medicine (DICOM). The DICOM standard is still under development, the latest release came out in June, 1994. It is expected that approval of this standard will be pursued via NEMA, which is accredited by ANSI, in the near future. ACR/NEMA has also published standards on magnetic tape and data compression. ACR/NEMA is working with AIIM to produce standards for of Picture-Archiving and Communication Systems (PACS). A discussion of the requirements of PACS to display radiological images is presented in the Storage and Transmission of Radiological Images.

American Society for Testing and Materials Committee E31 (ASTM E31)

ASTM E31 is a committee administered by ASTM charged with the development of healthcare informatics standards. Most of its work is in the form of draft standards dealing with the transfer of messages between clinical laboratory instruments and computer systems. In the area of data content, the draft of the ASTM E1384-91, dated October 29, 1993, titled "Standard Guide for the Description of Content and Structure of an Automated Primary Record of Care" is considered a good starting point as a basis for discussion. It is expected that ASTM will seek accreditation of these standards by ANSI on a selective basis when they are ready. There are six ASTM subcommittees that deal with standards that are relevant to the computer-based patient medical record. The ASTM E33.11 subcommittee publishes the E1238-88 standard which focuses on the transmission of clinical laboratory results [ASTM, 1993]. HL7 has worked closely over the years with the American Society for Testing Materials (ASTM) and with the exception of some minor differences (resulting from separate revision schedules) the ASTM and HL7 standard specifications are identical. E1238-88 can be used for the exchange of diagnostic orders and patient observations, including clinical laboratory, admission and discharge notes, electrocardiograms, consultation notes, etc.

Health Level 7 (HL7)

HL7 is an organisation developing standards for healthcare informatics dealing primarily with intra-hospital medical data transfers. It is an application protocol. HL7 is so named because it deals with data transfers at the OSI application layer—Layer 7 — for electronic exchange in healthcare environments. Its documents are expected to be submitted for approval as American National Standards Institute as well when they are considered ready. Again, HL7 standards development activities are very important to the development of EDI within the healthcare industry. Therefore, we devote an entire section on HL7 later in this chapter.

Institute of Electrical and Electronics Engineers (IEEE)

IEEE is a large professional organisation which is currently developing several standards of specific interest to the healthcare informatics community to be subsequently submitted for approval as American National Standards. Two IEEE committees, the IEEE Medical Data Interchange

(MEDIX) and the Medical Information Bus (MIB) committees have taken the lead in the development of standards documents for healthcare informatics. As a particular example, the IEEE Draft P1073 specifies standards for medical device communications [IEEE, 1994]. MEDIX is also very important to the development of EDI in clinical applications. For this reason, we provide a section on MEDIX later in this chapter.

Association for Information and Image Management (AIIM)

AIIM is a professional vendor oriented organisation carrying out standards development primarily in the area of data transfer and integrity in document imaging. Two of their published standards are:

Part 1: Performance Guidelines for the Admissibility of Records Produced by Information Technology Systems as Evidence, ANSI/AIIM TR31 (1993), and

Part 2: Performance Guidelines for the Legal Acceptance of Records Produced by Information Technology Systems.

Imaging and image transfer are major issues in the development of EDI but this field is plagued with technical aspects. Both system design analysts and medical and administrative professionals have concerns about the quality of computerized images and the integrity of the received image compared with the transmitted image. The HINT team decided to investigate the system design characteristics of these systems and the results of this investigation.

National Council for Prescription Drug Programmes (NCPDP)

NCPDP is an organisation developing standards for healthcare informatics specifically related to the prescription drug and pharmacy community. It is expected that the resulting documents will be submitted to ANSI for accreditation as national standards upon completion of the work. Interestingly, the pharmacy community is already operating with extensive EDI applications. "De facto" standards exist instituted by pharmaceutical manufacturers and wholesalers although most of the standards tend to have proprietary elements to them and therefore represent WANs rather than open system, national networks. Linking pharmacies to other entities in the healthcare community requires changes in these WANs so they can send and receive on a full industry wide EDI network.

Medical Terminology Standards

Codes representing various medical terminology are published by the following organisations:

- — American Dental Association (ADA)
- — American Medical Association (AMA)
- — Health Care Financing Administration (HCFA)
- — Health Insurance Association of America (HIAA)
- — National Center for Health Statistics
- — National Uniform Billing Committee (NUBC)
- — Superintendent of Documents, U.S. Government Printing Office

Needless to say, these codes are not uniform among all the organisations thereby leading to the compatibility problems discussed earlier in this chapter.

American Dental Association (ADA)

ADA's efforts to develop healthcare informatics standards are quite recent. ADA is also accredited by ANSI to submit documents that it develops for recognition as American National Standards. The ADA publishes the American Dental Association Journal. The journal contain the American Dental Association's codes for dental procedures and nomenclature and is the professionally recognised set of numeric codes for reporting dental treatments.

American Medical Association (AMA)

The AMA publishes the Current Procedural Terminology (CPT-4) Manual. The manual is a listing of descriptive terms and identifying codes for reporting medical services and procedures performed by Physicians. Examples of CPT-4 codes are:

- 33502 Anomalous coronary artery: ligation
- 33503 Anomalous coronary artery: graft w/o bypass
- 33504 Anomalous coronary artery: graft w/ bypass
- 33511 Coronary artery bypass, autogenous graft; 2 grafts

Health Care Financing Administration (HCFA)

HCFA publishes several documents containing standard healthcare codes. Among them are the:

- Health Care Financing Administration Common Procedural Coding System is a coding scheme to organise procedures performed into groups that are referenced for payment to providers.
- Health Care Financing Administration Code Lists is a coding scheme to document providers.
- Electronic Media Claims National Standard Format, is a variety of codes indicating the place where service was rendered.

These three documents form the basis for the submission of health care claims under the UB-92 Electronic Claims Standards.

Health Insurance Association of America (HIAA)

The Health Insurance Association of America publishes the National Healthcare Claim Payment Advice Committee Bulletins. The bulletins describe standard codes and messages that detail the reason why an adjustment was made to a healthcare claim payment by the payer. HIAA also publishes the National Insurance Codes, a series of bulletins that describe a series of codes used in electronic standards by the insurance industry.

National Center for Health Statistics

The National Center for Health Statistics publishes the International Classification of Diseases, 9th Revision, Clinical Modification (ICD-9-CM). ICD-9-CM describes the classification of morbidity and mortality information for statistical purposes and for the indexing of hospital records by disease and operations. Examples of ICD-9-CM codes are:

— 410 Acute myocardial infarction
— 410.0 Acute myocardial infarction of anterior wall
— 410.1 Acute myocardial infarction of other anterior wall
— 412 Old myocardial infarction

The ICD code in combination with the CPT code is accepted by many payers to identify the medical reason for treatment and the treatment administered.

National Uniform Billing Committee (NUBC)

NUBC publishes the National Uniform Billing Data Element Specifications. Among these specification are:

— Revenue codes (UB82 and UB92) which classify hospital charges in a standard grouping that is controlled by the National Uniform Billing Committee.
— Admission Source Code explaining who recommended admission to a medical facility.
— Admission Type Code explaining the priority of the admission to a medical facility.
— Claim Frequency Type Code explaining the frequency of the bill submission.
— Uniform Billing Claim Form Bill Type describing the type of medical facility.

— Patient Status Code indicating the patient status as of the statement covers through date.

Superintendent of Documents, U.S. Government Printing Office

The Superintendent of Documents, U.S. Government Printing Office, publishes the Federal Register and Health Insurance Manual 15 (HIM 15). This manual establishes the Diagnosis Related Group Number (DRG). The DRG is a patient classification scheme that clusters patients into categories on the basis of the patient's illness, diseases and medical problems.

Detailed Information On Standard Setting Groups

As noted in the previous section, four standards setting groups are particularly important to the development of EDI in the healthcare industry. Most of these standards are defined at the OSI layer seven, applications. These will be described in the next four sections. We begin with ANS X12.

American National Standard X12

ANS X12 does not deal specifically with healthcare data, but instead deals with the transfer of a wide variety of business related data. For example, nearly all credit card and bank card transactions in the U.S. are governed by X12 standard protocols. Therefore, the ANS X12 standard seems a natural umbrella for the administrative activities in the healthcare industry. In 1979, the American National Standards Institute (ANSI) chartered the Accredited Standards Committee (ASC) X12 to develop uniform standards for inter-industry electronic interchange of business transactions [DISA, 1991]. The main objective of the ASC X12 committee is to develop standards to facilitate electronic interchange relating to such business transactions as order placement and processing, shipping and receiving, invoicing, and payment and cash application data. X12 defines EDI as the transmission in a standard syntax, of unambiguous information of business or strategic significance between computers of independent organisations.

In November 1991, the Workgroup for Electronic Data Interchange (WEDI) was established in response to the challenge to reduce administrative costs in the nation's healthcare system. Recently, ASC X12 recognised WEDI as the organisation responsible for developing EDI transactions for the healthcare industry. X12 has approved some of the standards developed by WEDI as noted in 3.2.4.2. There are more than 20 standards in various stages of development and use which have applicability to health care. Currently several specific healthcare standards are classified as "Draft Standards for Trial Use" (DT) or "In Development" (ID) while other are in the formative stages and unclassified.

Transaction 270 - Healthcare Eligibility / Benefit Inquiry

This transaction set can be used to inquire about healthcare eligibility and benefits associated with a subscriber or a dependent under the subscriber's policy. A subscriber is a person who elects the benefits and is affiliated with the payer (insurer, HMO, etc.). A dependent is a person who is affiliated with the subscriber such as spouse, child, etc., and therefore may be entitled to benefits.

An example of the overall structure of the 270 Transaction Set is:

— Eligibility or Benefit Information Source
— Eligibility or Benefit Information Receiver
— Subscriber
— Dependent
— Eligibility or Benefit Inquiry (Question)
— Eligibility or Benefit Inquiry (Question)

As the paragraph above indicates, the transaction is specific between one provider and one payer. It deals with only one subscriber and/or one dependent (may be the subscriber), but may contain several questions. Typically, as a patient enters a providers service facility, the provider wants to know who is paying for the services requested. If the patient attests to a third party payer, the provider wants to confirm the payer's responsibility and the extent of that responsibility at the time of service delivery. This 270 transaction is designed to initiate this function for the provider. Nearly all physicians and most hospitals use telephone inquiries to payers. Telephone inquiries require person to person interaction where both humans use their time to interchange information and both may be referring to computer terminals to "obtain" and "read" and then "voice" transmit information. This is an inefficient use of human labor. The 270 EDI transaction takes place with a person initiating a computerized inquiry and a computer responding.

Transaction 271 - Healthcare Eligibility / Benefit Information

This transaction set can be used to communicate from healthcare information sources (i.e., insurers, sponsors, payers, etc.) to healthcare information receivers (i.e., physicians, hospitals, medical facilities, etc.) information about healthcare eligibility or benefits. This information includes but is not limited to: benefit status, explanation of benefit status, dependent coverage level, dates of coverage, covered days and/or non-covered days, amounts for co-insurance, co-pays, deductibles, exclusions and limitations. An example of the overall structure of the 271 Transaction Set is:

— Eligibility or Benefit Information Source
— Eligibility or Benefit Information Receiver
— Subscriber

- Eligibility or Benefit Information (Answer)
- Subscriber
- Dependent
- Eligibility or Benefit Information (Answer)
- Eligibility or Benefit Information (Answer)

As the paragraph above indicates, the transaction is specific between one payer(source) and one provider(receiver), but may contain numerous subscribers and/or dependents and several answers. The idea is that although each request is for an individual patient, the information source could answer multiple questions within a single reply message. Perhaps it goes without saying that this transaction is the detailed response to the inquiry initiated by the 270 transaction. The paired transactions, 270 and 271, eliminates a person to person telephone call replacing it with a computer to computer EDI interchange and provides an electronic record of the answer.

Transaction 278 - Healthcare Services Review Information

This transaction set can be used to transmit healthcare service information, such as patient, demographic, diagnosis or treatment data for the purpose of notification, or reporting the outcome of a healthcare services review. Expected users of this transaction set are payers, plan sponsors, providers, utilisation management, government agencies and/or other entities involved in healthcare services review. Basically the transaction is designed to provide for interested (and authorized) parties to make inquiry into the EDI system to obtain healthcare information that will be used for a variety of worthwhile purposes. Certainly, the EDI system will be used to periodically produce reports on the status of healthcare services, frequency of patient illnesses, etc., that are necessary to assure the quality of healthcare in society.

Transaction 834 - Benefit Enrollment and Maintenance

This transaction set can be used to establish communication between the sponsor of the health benefit product and the payer. Such transaction(s) may or may not take place through a third party administrator (TPA). For the purpose of this standard, the sponsor is the party or entity that ultimately pays for the benefit coverage or product. A sponsor can be an employer, labor union, government agency, association, or insurance agency. It is unlikely that individuals purchasing health benefits solely for themselves would use this transaction, but it is possible that such purchases may move through a healthcare alliance or other organisation that would use this transaction. The payer refers to an entity that pays claims, administers the insurance product or benefit, or both. A payer can be an insurance company, health maintenance organisation (HMO), preferred provider organisation (PPO), government agency (Medicare, Medicaid, Champus, etc.), or third party administrator that pays claims on behalf of another organisation such as one of the previous entities. For the purpose of the 834 transaction set, a third party administrator (TPA) can be contracted by a sponsor to handle data gathering from those covered by the sponsor if the sponsor does not elect to perform this function itself. Regardless of the entities involved, this transaction allows the two entities—sponsor and administrator—to exchange information about the subscribers and their dependents. Administrators need this information to be able to pay providers. For sponsors with large numbers of subscribers, initial enrollment and enrollment changes can be the source of large numbers of transactions. New Jersey based, AT&T Corporation became a national leader in 834 implementation by recently testing implementing this transaction for its employees with its third party administrators. We provide a detailed description of this pilot test (now aN accepted procedure for AT&T enrollments).

Transaction 835 - Healthcare Claim Payment/Advice

This transaction set can be used to make a payment, send an explanation of benefits (EOB) remittance advice, or make a payment and send an EOB remittance advice from a payer to a provider either directly or via a financial institution. This 835 can be sent only from a payer to a provider. When electronic funds transfers become common place among payers and providers, it will be necessary for payers to advise providers as to those claims that have been paid by the fund transfers. This is necessary so that providers can make the appropriate entries in their internal accounting system.

Transaction 837 - Healthcare Claim

This transaction standard is to be used to submit heath care claim billing information from providers to payers, either directly or via intermediary billers and/or claims clearinghouses. It can also be used to transmit heath care claims and billing payment information between payers with different payment responsibilities where coordination of benefits is required.

For purposes of this standard, providers of heath care products or services may include a wide variety of entities such as physicians, hospitals and other medical facilities or suppliers, dentists, and pharmacies. In some instances, more than one payer has responsibility for payment of the claim. For example, Medicare eligible patients frequently have additional "insurance" to pay for services not covered in part or total by Medicare. This situation creates a need for a "coordination of benefits" (COB) transaction so that the claim payment responsibility can be divided and sent to the separate payers. No such transaction set presently exists. However, work is underway to determine whether COB can be incorporated into the existing 837 claims transaction or whether a new transaction will be needed. Currently all

COB claims are the responsibility of the provider and/or patient. Claims transactions are so numerous (over one billion in 1992) and so important to the financial viability of the healthcare system that they dominate all other transactions. For that reason, we provide a detailed description of the 837 transaction set in the following paragraphs. This description includes claim details and notes explaining the usage of the various loops and segments. It has been proposed that the Segment ID be common throughout all X12 transactions. However the order of the segments, required use thereof (M = mandatory, O = optional) and the maximum use are unique to each ANS X12 numbered transaction.

Transaction 864 - Text Message

Not infrequently, users of an EDI system send messages to each other including messages about claims. This text message transaction standard can be used to provide users with a capability to electronically move messages, or other text such as contracts. This would be unique text material that does not fit into a standard predefined format as expected for claims, benefit inquiries, etc. It is the intent of this transaction set to provide electronic communication (messages) for people to read rather than for computer processing. The use of the transaction set to transmit quasi or unique transaction set standards is discouraged.

The use of the text message transaction set demands the sender provide certain detailed information about the recipient, specifically a mail address. The transaction set's purpose is to provide communication to the recipient in some human-readable form. The recipient's network will dictate what capabilities are available for delivery of the information. It is the responsibility of the sender to obtain this information and include it in the transmission.

Sample X12 Transaction (Subset)

Every 837 transaction will carry a specific, predefined quantity of information. The following paragraphs explain what information is defined and gives an example of the information that could be included. A description of the actual transaction is provided at the end of this section.

Summary of ANS X12

These transactions constitute those that have received ASC X12 approval as standards. That they are critically important is evident in the fact that effective May 1, 1994, HCFA required the 837 as the standard for electronic transmission of claims to Medicare. Eventually, it is expected that HCFA will require all claims to be submitted electronically using the X12 837 standard. Thus, HCFA has taken the first federal government steps towards standards for EDI.

Health Level 7

Health Level 7 (HL7) is a health-care specific, application level protocol which has been developed by an ad hoc organisation consisting of hospital, vendor and consultant volunteers. Initial efforts began in March of 1987 and continue to date The current version addresses interfaces for admissions, discharges, and transfers (ADT), clinical instructions, lab results, patient observation records, charges and other billing data. Of the four major healthcare data exchange standards, it has the widest scope and is the most widely used data exchange standard. The current trend in the HL7 organisation is to develop the standard in a less ad hoc manner and to adopt techniques that will direct the standard in a more deliberate manner with the goal of developing a more stable and robust standard [Perl, 1994]. On June 17, 1994 the ANSI regulatory authority formally recognised the HL7 organisation as an approved ANSI standard committee [Helath Level Seven, 1994]. HL7 has emerged as a major factor in standards for clinical information. Although it primarily has been focused on intra-provider (especially hospitals) communications, the standards can be modified to work in EDI. Thus, HL7 is an important standard for the future of clinical data transmission via EDI.

HL7 Description

HL7 is a standard for electronic medical data exchange in healthcare environments, with special emphasis on hospitals. It should be noted that HL7 takes its name from but does not conform to the ISO defined elements of the OSI's seventh layer. However, it does conform to the conceptual definition of an application to application interface protocol. HL7 as an application protocol specifies the data to be exchanged, the timing of the exchanges, and the communication of certain application specific errors between applications. Sensing the need to supply assistance to developers who do not operate in a complete OSI environment, the standard also specifies a set of encoding rules. These rules constitute the transfer syntax which is a function of the OSI level 6 or presentation layer. The standards allow for unique, or proprietary arrangements to exist between any two communicators. Thus, the standards do not automatically assure open network of communications as the layer 6 and 7 protocols on some LANs and WANs can be different than on others. Currently, the HL7 standard specifies the structure of interfaces for:

- Admission, discharge, transfer and registration
- Order entry
- Generalized querying
- Patient accounting systems
- Ancillary data, such as laboratory results.

There are numerous other areas under development, including:

— Master files operations (query and update)
— General financial systems
— Insurance billing
— Scheduling
— Additional detail for specific ancillary departments
— Nursing applications.

The HL7 design is based on a set of general goals. The first goal is that it be practical, which to the developers of HL7 means that it should be usable in a wide range of environments, from a full seven level OSI environment to less complete environments, such as a simple standard electronic cable connection. The second goal is that the standard should accommodate site specific variations. This has been accomplished by allowing sites to create their own message types and record definitions. The third goal is to support evolutionary growth. This capability has been built in by requiring that changes to the record definitions be made only by adding fields and never by deleting. The fourth major goal is to be supportive rather than prescriptive. While this goal is less easily identifiable in the specification, it is an important philosophy that is absolutely necessary in the very heterogeneous healthcare computing environment.

Applications communicate by transferring messages. The message is the smallest unit of data transferred between systems. In concept, the HL7 message is similar to the ANS X12 transactions explainedin this study The messages (transactions) are conceptually defined in terms of types that are named in terms of "trigger events," the real world events that initiate the exchange of messages. For example, admitting a patient to a hospital is a trigger event that defines an "admission" type message. Every message has a message type. A segment is a logical grouping of data items (fields) within a message. Each segment is given a name, for example ADT (Admission, Discharge, Transfer). The data items that compose the segments each have a name, a semantic description (meaning), a maximum length, a data type, optionally, and a note defining whether it can repeat. The HL7 data types are: string (ST), text (TX), formatted text (FT), numeric (NM), date (DT), time (TM), time stamp (TS), person name (PN), telephone number (TN), address (AD), coded value (ID), sequence ID (SI) and composite (CM, CK, CE, CQ). Composite data types consists of combinations of other meaningful data items. This data type can be used to transfer coded terms where it is necessary to also send the text description of the code and the name of the coding schema used. For example, using ICD-9CM coding schema we could send the code for brain neoplasm's as:

239.6^brain neoplasms NOS^ICD-9CM2

HL7 Transaction Checklist (excerpt)

The message transaction checklist documents the trigger events and messages defined by the HL7 standard. The checklist contains: a cover sheet describing the products being interfaced and the general characteristics of the interface, a message checklist to help establish which HL7 transactions will be used in the interface, who will be the originator of each message, the required and optional segments that will be sent in each of the messages, and a detailed list of all HL7 segment types identifying, by item:

- — sequence number,
- — item number,
- — field name,
- — required field indicator or place holder for selecting optional fields,

— data type,
— field length,
— maximum used,
— maximum allowable,
— repeating field indicator or place holder for maximum number of repetitions,
— variable name assigned to field on the sending system,
— variable name of field on the receiving system,
— table number (if applicable), and
— notes.

The checklist can be used during the development of an HL7 interface application. Once the hospital's data flow needs are established, the appropriate HL7 transactions can be selected from the checklist. Each transaction can be reviewed to determine which of the optional items will be included in the message (the required field which must be included in the message are already marked with an "R"). Descriptive information about the item (e.g., maximum character length, repeating/non-repeating field, type of time/ date notation, etc.) can be determined and documented on the checklist. The checklist also provides space to document the variable names assigned to corresponding fields on each system.

A checklist and cover sheet should be completed for each application interface being designed, including interfaces that broadcast to more than one system. In the case of broadcast interfaces, every effort should be made to agree on a single format for the message from the sender. Messages may include different segments and items, depending on the trigger event (e.g., pharmacy orders and lab orders both use the same message). Complete copies of the message selection/definition documentation for each trigger event should be prepared and filed. This level of specification is suitable for using the HL7 Standard in environments that implement up to the presentation and other high level services. The system application programmer would simply fill in the necessary data elements in the various segments and let the lower level services encode the message into the transfer syntax and transport the message to the receiving application. However, in an environment that does not have a OSI presentation layer, but does have at least a robust OSI transport layer, the HL7 Standard specifies a set of encoding rules that can be used.

HL7 Interface Checklist Cover Sheet

When setting up HL7 messages, the HL7 committee recommends that a checklist be produced so that the message syntax is clearly understood by both (could be three or more) systems. A typical check list looks like that below. The first section describes the interface between two users. System "A" and "B" are used to designate the sender and receiver in the message checklist section of the document.

Describing the interface between:

System A:

System B:

Checklist completed on: _____/_____ /_____.

Agreed to by: _________________________ and _________________________.

HL7 Messages

As described above, the HL7 standard for EDI transactions is based on messages. HL7 messages are currently clustered into six groups. The six groups are composed of messages that contain similar information, e.g. Admission, Discharge and Transfer Messages. Each message (e.g. Admit a Patient) is then broken into individual segments (i.e. Message Header, Event Type, Patient ID, Next of Kin, etc.). The segments are then defined by Items (which are nominally fields). However, Items may consist of one or more components (individual fields) as in the case of the Patient Address item which includes street address, city, state and zip code. The six currently defined message groups are:

Control Section

ACK - General Acknowledgment

MCF - Delayed Acknowledgment

Admission, Discharge and Transfer Messages

A01 - Admit a Patient
A02 - Transfer
A03 - Discharge
A04 - Register a Patient
A05 - Pre-Admit a Patient
A06 - Transfer Outpatient-Inpatient
A07 - Transfer Inpatient-Outpatient
A08 - Update Patient Information
A09 - Patient Departing
A10 - Patient Arriving
A11 - Cancel Admit
A12 - Cancel Transfer
A13 - Cancel Discharge
A14 - Pending Admit
A15 - Pending Transfer
A16 - Pending Discharge
A17 - Swap Patients
A18 - Merge Patient Information
A19 - Patient Query
A20 - Nursing/Census Updates

A21 - Patient Out on LOA
A22 - Patient Returns from LOA
A23 - Delete a Patient Record
A24 - Create a Patient Link

3.4.4.3 Order Messages

ORM - Order Message
ORR - Order Response

3.4.4.4 Queries

Q01 - Query for Immediate Response
Q03 - Query for Deferred Response
Q05 - Unsolicited Updates

3.4.4.5 Finance: Patient Accounting

P01 - Add/Update Patient Accounts
P02 - Purge Patient Accounts
P03 - Detail Financial Transaction

3.4.4.6 Ancillary Data Reporting

ORU - Unsolicited Observation
ORF - Observational Report

HL7 Message Segments

Messages are composed of segments. Each segment contains a series of Items (fields or series of fields). Segments may be used in more that one message. For example, the Patient Identification (PID) is required in most messages.

ADD - Addendum
BHS - Batch Header
BLG - Billing
BTS - Batch Trailer
DG1 - Diagnosis Information
DSC - Continuation Pointer

DSP - Display Data
ERR - Error
EVN - Event Type
FHS - File Header
FT1 - Financial Transaction
FTS - File Trailer
GT1 - Guarantor
IN1 - Insurance
MRG - Merge Patient Information
MSA - Message Acknowledgment
MSH - Message Header
NK1 - Next of Kin
NTE - Notes and Comments
OBR - Observation Request
OBX - Result
ORC - Common Order
ORO - Order Other
PID - Patient Identification
PR1 - Procedures
PV1 - Patient Visit
QRD - Query Definition
QRF - Query Filter
RX1 - Pharmacy Order
UB1 - UB82 Data
URD - Results/Update Definitions
URS - Unsolicited Selection
Z - Z segment (hospital specific)

A01 - Admit a Patient - Message Detail

The following paragraphs provide a example of a detailed message. We have selected the "Admit a Patient" message as typical of HL7. The message segments are shown below.

Note that the first five segments are required while the last two are optional. The `Z', hospital specific segment, is optional. Multiple `Z' segments can be mutually defined for data exchange between `System A' and `System B' using any three character segment ID beginning with the letter `Z'.

Details of the first four individual segments are shown below with their Items in sequence order. Just as some segments of a message are optional, so are some items within a segment. Notice that the message segments are defined by event that triggers the message. First is the necessary message header and event type, next are the segments associated with the particular trigger event, in this case Patient Admission.

Message Segment Summary

One additional segment, patient visit, is required in this message. Two others are available but not required, diagnosis information and hospital specific information. These are not shown here because they are very lengthy and would add little additional understanding to this exposition of detail. What is important is the complexity of detail that this somewhat routine event requires in terms of computer definitions and standards. This is the critical link between application design and reality. This can be further understood by providing a sample message that demonstrates the characters that are actually transmitted across the line from one user to another.

HL7 Sample Message

The message formats prescribed in the HL7 encoding rules consist of data items that are of variable length and separated by a item separator character. The rules describe how the various data types are encoded within a field and when an individual field may be repeated. The data fields are combined into logical groupings called segments.

Segments are separated by the segment separator character, i.e. the ASCII Carriage Return character '<cr>'. Each segment begins with a three-character literal value that identifies it within a message. Segments may be defined as required or optional, and may be permitted to repeat. Individual data items are found in the message by their position with their associated segments. When a data item is empty, an item separator (usually the ASCII Vertical Bar character '|') marks its position. When an Item contains multiple included components (individual fields), they are separated by the component separator (usually the ASCII Tilde character '~'). All data is represented by displayable ASCII characters. All the special separators and other special characters are also displayable ASCII characters, except that the segment separator is the ASCII Carriage Return character '<cr>'. Sample data is shown below for the five required segments of the patient admit message "A01" described in the previous section. Multiple optional segments are left blank here to avoid additional detail.

This is the actual string of characters that would be sent from one computer to another. Using the services of the OSI level 5 (Session) or the equivalent in a non-OSI environment, e.g. file transfer, IBM LU6.2, TCP/IP sockets or SUN RPC, this character string can be transmitted to the receiving application. The receiving system will use level 6 type services to convert the encoded string into an abstract message structure and then extract data fields as needed by the application (level 7). The standards also specify an acknowledgment protocol so that the sending application can determine whether the data was received exactly as sent. This example exemplifies the complexity that makes message composition and transmission difficult. And, this complexity exists even when standards are present. Without standards, messages transmitted with complete clarity by one machine are received as a jumble of unintelligible characters by another machine operating with a different standard.

CASE STUDY: MANAGEMENT INFORMATION SYSTEMS AND THE USE OF COMPUTERS IN UK HOSPITALS

The concept of Management Information has developed over many years but it has always been necessary for any organisation to acquire information in order to be aware of its own state, and the state, of its environment, particularly that of its 'market', including the potential and strategy of its competitors. This is most vividly illustrated in the realm of military intelligence. The use of such information (and misinformation) has played a crucial part in every military campaign and increasingly so in recent times, no doubt due to our growing, capability to acquire and use it. We now recognise this capacity with a particular designation—Information Technology (IT) and the integ-ration of IT into the management of an enterprise as Management Information Systems (MIS). In the NHS these concepts underpin the Korner reports on NHS management information which call not only for new data acquisitions to be made but also for an integration of the MIS with organisational requirements at all levels of the service. The requirements and effects of Korner will be examined in detail later in the chapter. It is, perhaps wise initially to look at and explain some of the concepts of systems theory.

Systems And Sub-Systems

First the term 'system' requires clarification. We frequently use this word in a wide social context when referring, for example, to the education system, the political system, or the social system itself. In doing so we accept that the particular components that make up each system exhibit a special significance within the system which they would not do independently. For example, there would be little point in admitting patients to hospital without the various diagnostic treat-ment and support systems being available. In turn each one of these systems is given relevance only by the presence of patients to care for.

One of the shortest definitions describes a system as 'a set of interrelated elements'. However, as illustrated by the health system, these elements may also comprise other systems—sub-systems—which are required to function in harmony with each other and with other components in order to attain the objectives of the organisation. This is particularly true of the health care system with its multiple objec-tives, disparate client demands and its many professionally dominated sub-systems and occupational groups. Systems theory has contributed to the development of concepts in sociology, economic analysis, engineering, management information, automation in general and improved technologies, management schools and so on. A system, then, may be regarded as any group of inter-related and interdependent entities or functions that combine for a specific pur-pose. In so doing a system receives certain inputs and is constrained to act concertedly upon them to produce certain outputs with the objec-tive of maximizing some function of the inputs and outputs. All systems appear to require at some time inputs of various kinds. These are known as open systems. The need for inputs makes them vulnerable to their environment. Closed systems on the other hand tend to exist only for finite intervals. A wrist watch may be regarded as a relatively closed system until it requires correcting or mending, winding or a new battery! A classification of systems types is discussed by Boulding.

A further systems clarification may be made to differentiate *determi-nistic* and *probabilistic* systems. A deterministic system is one in which the parts interact in a perfectly predictable way. A probabilistic system on the other hand is one about which no precise detailed prediction can be given. Many problems occur because the same systems are regarded by some people as deterministic and by others as probabilis-tic. For example, once a patient's name is placed on a hospital waiting list, eventually they will be notified that a bed is available. This might be regarded as a deterministic sub-system in the waiting list admissions process. However, on the day there may be no bed available or the patient may fail to attend and the system may be seen as probabilistic

When we apply this analysis to the health care system we are confronted with an enormous organisation with a great many elements and sub-systems and not a few objectives, although it could be argued that some boundaries are self-determining. Our next problem is to identify where these occur or could be appropriately defined.

Systems Boundary

This problem is of particular interest in the NHS since the reorganisa-dons of 1974 and 1982 have sought to shift systems boundaries with consequent changes in status and morale for all concerned. If we accept with Crowe and Avison that 'the organisation itself is the correct boundary for the system' then that still leaves us the task of defining the term 'organisation' within the NHS. For practical purposes we believe we may take this to be the lowest level of organisation that is independently accountable to statutory authority, i.e. the District Health Authority. The district, although itself a sub-system in the regional and national health system, would perceive these 'external entities as forming part of its environment and would regard every sub system as a subordinate contributor in the optimization process. Such a view would seem to accord with the present management and accountability structure. Past organisational structures either made the systems boundaries too small (Hospital Board) or unman-ageably large (Area Health Authorities). The result was that each organisational entity tended to perform independently. The necessity for management information required by the organisation was poorly perceived by hospital departments and therefore poorly collected Local operational information requirements were collected on an ad *hoc* basis. Organisationally there arose 'no-go' areas with regard to management information. Standard returns were completed by local sub-system personnel, were limited in scope, and could be of varying accuracy. The current trend, however, is towards the integration of district information.

Stakeholders

A concept that requires clarification is that of stakeholding in a particular system or sub-system. A stakeholder is anyone who has an interest or stake in the system whether as a provider or a direct or indirect user of the system. Of course the degree of stakeholding can vary, for example:

- — a clinician seeking an X-ray for a patient
- — a hospital porter who takes the patient to the X-ray department
- — the patient being X-rayed
- — the radiographer, radiologist and the report typist.

All these, and others, are stakeholders to a greater or lesser degree in the radiology sub-system. Notice that this sub-system is not confined to the radiology department

It may be argued that the porter's interest in the radiology sub system is slight, yet, like everyone else employed in health care, he will hold a small stakeholding in many other sub-systems and principally in the hospital portering sub-system. The patient, on the other hand, will have a substantial stakeholding in every sub-system concerning his/her welfare, whereas the clinician may be expected to have a particular interest in those sub-systems which deal specifically with information flow. He will not usually be concerned to know what X-ray exposure interval was employed by the radiographer or the type of work processor used by the typist, but will be most concerned to receive the typed report and to learn its contents. The sub-system for returning the report, internal post, special delivery, or computer communications system, will concern the clinician, but often less so the service depart-ment once the report has been issued. It is impossible to obtain 100% commitment from workers in any single sub-system who themselves also have responsibilities in several other sub-systems. For this reason amongst others it is frequently difficult to reach unanimity amongst workers regarding sub-system goals and priorities.

Organisational Goals

Problems of organisational goal incongruence have been well discussed by Fox Simon and Ansoff, Simon and Cyert and March amongst many others. We merely note here that conflict may and does occur for a variety of reasons within sub-systems, particularly where these cross departmental boundaries, or where there is a clash of professional influence and opinion.

Much will depend upon the nature of the psychological contract that exists between individual workers and the organisation in which they are employed and whether the sub-systems in which they are involved meet their needs and provide them with motivation and satisfaction at work. Sub-system changes, therefore, potentially threaten this contrac-tual equilibrium and, unless such changes bring perceived improve-ments for workers, they will be resisted to some extent and ways will be sought to circumvent or avoid them. The manager's ability to manage change effectively will also be tested in these circumstances.

Management information systems are not exempt from these prin-ciples and where MIS imposition creates a requirement for a signifi-cant change in working practice their value will tend to be discounted or ignored by workers unless they bring tangible rewards. An example of this is to be found in the changes made to certain records which facilitate the free and necessary flow of highly personal information between patient and clinician. Lack of confidence in the security of this information may inhibit the consultation process. In these circum-stances clinicians may, individually or corporately, resist the system change and by-pass or ignore the computer in order to reassert their own professionalism. This particular problem is further compounded by the specific requirements of the 1985 Data Protection Act, although at the time of writing the relationship between the Act and medical (as opposed to personal) data is unclear. We return to the matter of confidentiality later in this study.

Organisations, on the other hand, are likely to react by a process of increased institutionalization, which may take a bureaucratic form, seeking to obtain compliance with its new requirements. Stakeholders may well respond by seeking to individualize their role, so as to optimize personal and/or professional goals in a trade-off with those of the organisation.

Systems And Environment

All open systems require inputs and produce outputs of some kind which are subject to environmental conditions. The introduction of cash limits, and the redistribution of health care funding through the RAWP formulae, may be regarded as examples of environmental constraints in the health service. Alternatively the freedom now enjoyed by health authorities to indulge in income generation is a similar 'environmental' change to which the health system as a whole is likely to react. Furthermore, developing patterns of health and disease will also exert pressure on the health care system. Social changes in such matters as smoking and drinking habits, the incidence of obesity, personal exercise patterns and diet will be reflected in the responding health care system. However, the predominant model of health care, the curative model, is strongly entrenched, and we expect to see resistance within the system to any change involving the transfer of money from the curative to the preventative model, which is not to say that the latter model might not be more desirable, efficient and cost-effective in certain circumstances.

The development of the disease AIDS, for example, has affected inputs, processes and outputs, i.e. the patients presenting for treat-ment, the additional resources utilized and the displacement of alterna-tive patients, are all system changes consequent to the environmental presence of Acquired Immune Deficiency Syndrome. Environmental, changes, then, are those which impose themselves and which the system has to deal with and adapt to.

Information

The systems concept is a fascinating one particularly when applied to information management. In all organisations there is a vast amount of data which is often mistaken for information. Data are indeed items of information, albeit unstructured and often unrelated. Information may be regarded simply as the meaning attached to data or struc-tured, organised and selected data with particular relevance to specific organisational or personal needs. It follows that the same set of data is capable of providing more than one piece of information depending on how the data are processed. Data processing has been defined as a systematic sequence of operations, performed on data with the object of extracting or revising information. Organisational decisions are based upon available information. In health care, however, there is a vast amount of 'information', particular larly of the unprocessed raw data variety which is untapped and is only now becoming available. As Kind and Prowle have said, every transaction between doctor and patient, every hospital admission and discharge, every payment to a health service employee generates one or more items of data. This is not to mention all the activity occurring as a consequence of these events. The reliability of information depends upon important factors such as:

— the quality of the raw data: a function of the data collection/ acquisition process
— the appropriateness of the data processing: selectivity the relative cost of obtaining the information
— the speed at which processed information is made available by the system.

Because the technology now exists, it is tempting to collect more data and to disseminate more information than ever before. However, Ackoff has identified five commonly held but mistaken assumptions about management information. These are:

1 More information is better than less—it is often too much.
3 Managers need what they ask for—they often ask for too much, or the wrong kind of information.
3. Decision-making will improve given the information—infor-mation is often ignored.
4. More communication means better performance—it may create conflict and make it worse.
5. Managers need only understand how to use the MIS—this does not mean that they *will* do so.

These false assumptions may help us to appreciate the management information/decision-making dilemma, particularly in large organisa-tions where data gathering is necessarily delegated and processed remotely from its source.

The Value of Information

Obviously, information possesses a value but little work has been attempted to identify it. Moreover, in general terms (except perhaps in trend analysis), information is most valuable immediately or shortly after the event to which it relates. Thereafter, it is likely to fall in value to both the individual and the organisations as the particular event is overtaken by fresh developments. This is well illustrated by clinical data following a clinical event such as a heart attack or diabetic instability where clinical information such as the result of a blood test will be most useful at the time of the event and will increasingly be only °f academic interest as time passes. There is a sense in which health care may be regarded as a datagathering and information processing system, since all health care activity follows the acquisition of clinical data from a variety of sources. This is distributed within the organisation by means of request and report forms, letters and patients' notes. The value and rate of decay of much of this clinical data is high, and its processing and communication, therefore, requires appropriate priority. While this has been recognised for clinical data the same view has not been generally extended to the management of the health care organisation itself and its particular information needs. It is clear that different stakeholders apportion different values to the same information. For example, clinicians will tend to regard a budget statement as a constraint and an irrelevance in meeting patient needs, whereas general managers will view budgets as instruments of control and each statement as an aid in overall resource management, ultimately for the good of the majority of patients. However, few managers at present are able to demonstrate the unit costs of medical and organisational activity or to identify quantitative measures of outcome of clinical treatment. The development of an appropriate MIS is an essential. prerequisite for improvements in these areas.

The Cost of Information

Separate retrospective data collection systems are costly, generally slow to yield information and tend to constrain the event system, for example, by requiring data documents such as request forms to remain available to the data collectors. If the task of separate data collection is given to a member of the event system the task value is easily discounted, badly performed or becomes displaced by alternative perceptions of priority. Should data collection become the responsi-bility of special data collection personnel, as in Hospital Activity Analysis, the error in collection may also be high. Data collectors may have low job satisfaction if they work solely with data items and are not concerned with their meaning. Other parts of the information jigsaw may be unavailable or of no significance to them. In addition, source documents may be mislaid, data access difficulties may arise and dependence upon the co-operation of others having a low stakeholding in the event system may all contribute to problems of accurate and reliable data collection.

However, we believe that data collection and information processing are factors of production, particularly in health care, that have been ignored for too long and the cost of adequate systems must now be faced. In the Korner recommendations there are staffing and techno-logical implications that can only be avoided at the expense of the very attributes and value of effective information systems we have outlined. The cost to the organisation of not collecting necessary data or of collecting it inadequately is high. We believe that in the long run it will prove to be higher than the cost of the necessary investment in appropriate management information systems.

Management Information Systems

Management information may be regarded as that information which relates directly or indirectly to the inputs, activities and outcomes of an organisation and its environment. Naturally, this will include all other systems which may and do interact with the organisation.

Information presents in a variety of ways. Hard facts such as non-staff costs may appear as invoices requiring payment. Staff costs are met through the salaries and wages payments. It is relatively simple to capture data on incurred expenditure using the departmental records of the finance department.

Outputs, on the other hand, have to do with the uses to which the health care system has been put and the goals attained thereby—illness prevention, preservation of life quality, and lives saved. These are difficult outcomes to measure and so proxy measures are frequently adopted. Such parameters as length of stay per specialty, bed occu-pancy, cost per case etc., may serve to indicate how financially efficient the health machine is as a closed system. They are unable to indicate the economic effectiveness of the system in terms of its primary objectives which relate to improved health outcomes for our popu-lation. We do not discount the value of activity indicators. As we shall see, they may be used to show where management scrutiny may be usefully applied; they have a role in any organisation. However, health out-comes measurement is also important, some would say vital, in any activity evaluation and is able and necessary to moderate the purely financial considerations of the health machine.

Present Regimes

The present mechanisms of gathering management information data within the NHS take the form of monthly returns, each designed to give a limited amount of specific information about an aspect of health care. Developments in the NHS have given rise to autonomous data collection systems, sometimes overlapping or even duplicating each other but, due to the specificity of purpose, being little use across the broad spectrum of health care management. Information for local needs has been largely displaced by the requirements of planners.

External Data Gathering

One of the ways that health information is obtained externally to the NHS is through the Office of Population Censuses and Surveya (OPCS) either by special surveys or through the General Household Survey. The General Household Survey is now carried out every other year. It consists of a comprehensive questionnaire put to households chosen at random. The questionnaire covers a wide range of infor-mation of which morbidity, self-treatment and the uptake of health services, for example, form but a part. Although incomplete, this information is probably the best regular evidence we receive about the nation's health and its needs, about individual behaviour in relation to health, and the effectiveness of our various health care provisions.

Internal Data Gathering

Information internal to the NHS, as we have seen, consists broadly of financial and non-financial data. Non-financial information regarding activity is summarized on Form SH3. The reliability of the source data for SH3 returns has been ques-tioned. There is no incentive for ward staff to be meticulous, since the information they collect is not generally perceived as useful to them. Moreover, there are difficult data collection problems to be overcome on busy wards. For example, classified beds (ones assigned to a particular specialty) are frequently temporarily shared between specialties as need arises. Then there are difficulties, some would say impossibilities, in stan-dardizing the classification of source data under every possible vari-ation from the assumed normal activity pattern. The problems are further compounded by the lack of a place to record readmissions, and the failure to differentiate between a death and discharge further reduces the potential usefulness of the information. In the past, SH3 data appears to have found little use at district level and, accordingly, its collection had low priority. Recently it has become apparent that such information will be required to support arguments concerning policy decisions and resource allocation. Once relevance has been shown, priority will undoubtedly increase.

Hospital Activity Analysis (HAA)

Hospital Activity Analysis (HAA) was introduced in 1969 and arose out of the perceived inadequacies of the Hospital Inpatient Enquiry,(HIPE). This system endeavoured to provide, by a process of sam-pling, information regarding inpatients, their illnesses and their oper-ations and to relate this information to notions of medical need in the community. HIPE is a manual data collection system and problems with sampling and excessive delays in reporting, together with the arrival of computers, gave rise to a further development: HAA. Hospital Activity Analysis is based upon the completion for every inpatient of a multipart form, HMR1. This form requests demo-graphic, preadmission, admission (and readmission) details with dates, including transfers between specialties. To these are added the princi-pal diagnosis, with underlying causes, principal operations and 'other investigations'. The date of discharge or death is also required.

These forms are completed by ward staff. Clinicians

are required to provide diagnostic information which is then computer encoded by HAA staff using the International Diagnostic Index. The top copy of the HMR1 form thus becomes a computer input document and is either forwarded to the regional computer or used locally where on-line facilities exist. The data captured in this was thought to be useful as a source of information for the clinicians regarding their activity and for medical research. Kind and Prowle found little evidence for this, rather that the clinicians themselves both discounted the value of HAA and in many cases declined for various reasons to co-operate fully in contributing to it. Nationally, there is no superimposition of quality control or data audit with HAA although some districts may attempt this. Although intended as a 100% sample survey, much lower sample rates have been reported, as have high error rates in the coding of diagnostic data.

The identification of cross-boundary flows, i.e. inpatients referred from outside a district or region who are of interest mainly to managers have proved to be about the most useful, though flawed statistic to have emerged from the HAA system. In truth the clinicians, ward clerks, nurses and indeed HAA staff are all low stakeholders in a system which demands from them an input, costly in terms of three time but which provides them with no concomitant rewards. No wonder that nearly 10 years after Kind and Prowle's research paper many clinicians still regard HAA data as 'rubbish'.

Sub-Disrict Returns

The activities of many departments in each district are returned on appropriate forms. The origins of the requirement for the requst information lie in the history of the evolved NHS management system from 1948 until the 1980s. Once again most activity information is filed centrally for planning purposes or used by finance departments to calculate crude unit costs for inclusion in the annual accounts. Such data is perceived by managements to be of little local value in managing a department, particularly one perceived as being demand led. Many staff are unaware of what data is returned or even of the information exercise itself. For reasons already discussed, errors in the initial data collection are high and vary between districts, thus reduc-ing the value of inter-district comparisons. Since no two districts are exactly alike, the value of these comparisons is doubtful in any case—a fact that has long been accepted. For example, a survey of pathology laboratories by Stenton revealed discrepancies in, and discussed problems of, data collections in these departments. Although the basic data definition is appended to the collection form (form SBH6),particular working practices and developments in pathology labora-tories, together with the general tendency to enhance departmental workload figures for resource allocation purposes, have, over the years, inflicted an aberration on the collected data which now renders it wholly unreliable. Indeed, we are aware of departments where proper data collection is regularly substituted by estimates based on data collected some 15 years previously and updated in proportion to current workload. We do not believe that every laboratory or even every department is as lax as in this example, but we would repeat that where activity information is of no significance to a department, that is to say it is perceived as an unnecessary feedback in systems management, the collection of data from which it is derived will be poorly disciplined and will require significant input of resources to improve. This will apply even if computers are used unless data can be acquired and processed automatically as a by-product of normal work.

Special Surveys

The inadequacies of early management information

gathering, as we have seen, lay fundamentally in the fact that its analysis and use occurred elsewhere than at its source. It could be argued that if early systems were unreliable and inflexible in their application, planners and managers who are concerned about reliability should conduct their own specific surveys rather than endeavour to abstract infor-mation from secondary and unreliable sources. To a certain extent the 1977-9 Royal Commission on the NHS with its many interviews, written evidence and research papers fulfilled that function for the government. Royal Commissions, however, are costly, and are not managerial processes.

Rayner Scrutinies

The emergence in the 1980s of a procedure known as the Rayner Scrutiny after its perpetrator, Lord Rayner, Chairman of Marks and Spencer, sought to fill this requirement. The procedure was developed in the context of the Civil Service where he was asked to identify waste and to recommend cost reduction methods and efficiency savings.

In the NHS, Rayner Scrutinies are carried out by a small team who examine one particular area with the above objectives in view. The examination period is usually short and intense. At the conclusion recommendations are anticipated. With the emphasis in these pro- cesses so heavily on cost reduction there is apprehension by NHS staff that quality of work will not be maintained or will be unacceptably reduced if the recommendations are accepted without fully considering the effects on service provision. The characteristics of goal-directed investigations operated from above is that they contribute nothing to integrated management information systems but act as a 'commando raid' on a narrow topic, plundering its information in a blinkered way to meet preset and specific objectives. They report and withdraw leaving managers who are now, by inference, guilty and must prove themselves innocent, having to provide a reason why they may not now make the savings recommended in the report. Of course we recognise that the way our service is delivered has to change and develop; that is axiomatic. If we are concerned about quality, however, should pure cost necessarily be our first axiom? When such norms are agreed and the service is clear about its objectives then we may set about fulfilling them as economically as possible within the agreed quality standards.

Performance Indicators

Performance indicators are statistics relating to the activities of various components or sections of health care within the NHS, presented in an accessible way and offered to managers as useful information. In a sense Pis merely make available to the operational level of the service in a regular, organised and ritual manner, information to which DHSS planners have long had access since it is derived from existing data collection systems such as SH3. PIs for specific service or client groups are based upon the recommendations of the Working Groups of the Joint Group on Per-formance Indicators (JGPI). Currently some 450 PIs have been de-scribed covering the work of the Acute, Support, Manpower, Estate Management, Mental Handicap, Mental Illness, Children and Elderly Working Groups. PIs are available in printed form or on floppy disc and may be obtained from the DHSS (Health Publications Unit, No. 2 Site, Manchester Road, Heywood, Lancashire OLIO 2PZ).

Use of PIs

The DHSS has stated that:

> 'PIs are intended to be practical and useful tools for management. They are indicators and not measures, as the name states. They provide pointers and signals

> to areas which appear to merit further investigation. They enable managers to make comparisons between the performance of their services and that of others throughout England. No PI should ever be used in isolation. No single PI or group of PIs will reveal conclusively whether performance is satisfactory or unsatisfactory. Average PI values should not be used as 'norms' or 'standards'. PIs provide a starting point for investigation. Local information, knowledge and experience are essential to assess the validity of inferences drawn from PIs.'

In spite of the above provisions, PIs have been criticized. They are capable of being applied coercively, particularly where money is scarce, to justify cuts at the expense of quality. For example, if we take, say, the PI, nursing and midwifery cost per case, if this were higher than average, the tendency might arise to reduce this without regard to the reasons for its original value. The central authorities' argument is that nurses, like any other health care profession, are probably bound to say that they cannot manage with fewer resources. Other criticisms have concerned the selection of particular PIs, poor data (PIs also rely on SH3 data) and their usefulness to medical and nursing staff. In 1984 a survey by Pollitt revealed that over half the 133 responding health authorities in England found PI data of little use. It is ironic that were PIs useful more trouble would be taken by users to collect the source data accurately, thus increasing their usefulness still further. One may expect general managers to address this problem particularly if they are themselves using this source of information.

A further criticism concerns the continuing absence of output indicators and measures of service quality, clinical effectiveness and patient satisfaction. It is in this sense that PIs could form, in due course, an integrated information system for managers, capable of indicating population need, the economic level of treatment, clinical outcomes and patient satisfaction. These last two Pollitt found con-sidered both desirable and possible by most health authorities. Some work has already begun on these matters.

Health Services Information —The Korner Reports

In 1980 the Secretary of State for Social Services appointed the NHS/ DHSS Steering Group on Health Services Information under the chairmanship of Mrs Edith Korner. The terms of reference were:

1. To agree, implement and keep under review principles and procedures to guide the future development of health services infor-mation systems.
2. To identify and resolve health service information issues requir-ing a co-ordinated approach.
3. To review existing health service information systems.
4. To consider proposals for changes to, or developments in, health service information systems arising elsewhere and, if acceptable, to assess priorities for their development and implementation.

In the first Korner report published in 1982 many inadequacies of the inherited NHS management information strategies were frankly acknowledged. The guiding principle adopted by the Steering Group was stated as being:

> '... an approach to the provision of information which is based on the requirement to collect data because they are essential for operational purposes: user-oriented infor-mation yields benefits to those who collect it, and thus provides an incentive for accuracy and expedition.'

A number of working groups were set up by the Steering

Group to investigate specific health service activities. All groups, however worked to the same pattern which is outlined in the *First Report*. The service activities specifically addressed were:

1. Hospital facilities used by consultant medical staff.
2. Laboratory and scientific services.
3. Paramedical services.
4. Community health services.
5. Health service manpower.
6. Health service management accounting.
7. Patient transport services.

Many sub-groups were set up to look at the detailed requirements these special areas.

The Steering Group also sought to address the problem that succe ful data collection does not automatically result in management information becoming available to, and being used by, health service managers. For example the reduction and management of waiting lists will be facilitated by the more comprehensive Korner data sets giving a detailed breakdown of people waiting for operations. The amount of time people have been on waiting lists will be more accurately known, as will the split between urgent and non-urgent cases. Thus the more organised approach to data management that Korner specifies will help 'front-line' staff to organise their work. But will they use and contribute to these facilities without training and motivation? Thus, part of the Steering Groups' task was conceived to be concerned with the training for both data collectors and information users, the development of data standards and the promotion of information technology. Since commencing work, the Korner Steering Group have produced their seven main reports together with supplementaries and a report on confidentiality. These have been accepted by the Secretary of State and the

Korner hospital-based information systems were scheduled for implementation in April 1987 with the community systems to follow a year later. One obvious change is that from these dates the 'statistical' year will become synonymous with the financial year.

Minimum Data Sets

Korner believes that it is possible to identify a minimum set of data for each sub-system which should be used in all districts and that the data should be collected largely as a by-product of operational procedures. In order to do this effectively, particularly in departments and sub-systems where computers are yet to be deployed, the minimum data set needs to be simple, easy to collect, and useful to local stakeholders as well as to district officers. Indeed Korner believes that where data are not locally useful it is unlikely to be of use at higher levels and there is therefore no point in collecting it. Information derived in this way is intended to permit valid inter-district comparisons to be made. At present these are attempted using Pis. This requirement highlights the need for improved data definitions and standard practices in making returns to be adopted throughout the NHS. Only as data collection becomes standardized and source data are consequently more reliable will improvements in management information become possible. Some managers will require more than the Korner minimum and they will have to balance desirability with feasibility and cost. It is likely that some requirements will be impossible to meet without the use of computer systems and this will obviously apply to the establish-ment of databases in the specified areas of health care. Changes in clinical practice and in district organisation may be expected to make iresh demands on the MIS; relevance and timeliness of data collection will require review. The MIS will facilitate adaptation to new requirements by having precise data definitions and an adequate database facility, so that information may be accurately acquired from the data in response to a variety of needs rather than to one specific requirement.

Problems With Korner Implementation

At the time of writing we are still awaiting the full implementation of Korner. In most districts Korner implementation officers have been appointed to review data collection systems and identify training needs. However, this task is enormous and different departments possess widely different data collection capabilities and attitudes Moreover, the implementation of Korner comes at a time when new computerized Patient Administration Systems (PAS) are being intro-duced to meet specific local needs, so that across the NHS as a whole quite different systems co-exist to handle essentially the same type of data. The Patient Administration System will eventually replace and supersede the existing HAA. It is also designed to streamline many others of the administrative procedures concerning patient manage-ment which are currently performed manually. However, implemen-tation is often modular and will therefore entail a considerable degree of overlap of systems until all modules of the PAS are installed.

Typically, the full PAS will comprise five modules. These are:

Patient Registration: used for maintaining a master index holding basic details for each patient coming into contact with in- or outpatient services in the district. Since other modules utilize information from this module, this will be the first module to be installed.

Inpatient system: monitors and records administrative informations arising from a patient's stay in hospital. This module will support the DIS (District Information System).

Outpatient module: will manage appointments for outpatient depart-ments, making appointments information readily available in different formats to support the administrative functions of those departments *Waiting list module:* will maintain waiting lists and provide infor-mation about all planned admissions.

District Information System: will replace existing HAA as a manage-ment information system providing patient-based data, including medical information.

There remains the fundamental problem of increasing the stakeholding of those who actually record source data: the nurses, ward clerks, office staff and so on. How important is it for them in the performance of their daily work that accurate information from the data they collect is fed back to them so that their tasks become easier, more interesting and more personally satisfying and they thus become fully committed to accurate data collection?

If departments have managed to exist until the present without better management information, will they know what to do with it if and when it becomes available? Of course, such a question ignores the fact of organisational development and change, which, as we have already seen, includes, for the NHS, plans for management budgeting and the cross-charging of clinical cost centres for work performed in service departments. This not only presupposes an efficient MIS but places an unacceptable strain on the Korner minimum data set. As an example, let us consider one such service department, pathology, for which Korner recommends that the minimum amount of data col-lected equals the number of requests received. The *First Report* made this recommendation 'with the clear understanding that health auth-orities will wish to collect additional data to describe the local situation if firm control arrangements are to be instituted and improved man-agement achieved'.

The report also recommended that research be commissioned into the development of cost control techniques that could be adopted easily by local management.

With clinical budgeting two data requirements are immediately obvious. It is clear that the source of each request, by specialty or individual clinician, will require collection. Secondly, it is equally obvious that while a 'request' is a clinical activity with certain oper-ational relevance, it is the tests performed by the pathology labora-tories in response to such requests that cause resources to be consumed and which therefore should be the basis for cross-charging. Not only may a single request imply one or several tests, but further laboratory work may automatically ensue from the results of the initially requested work. Resource implications of requested work vary widely and as we have seen may depend upon the time at which the request is made. The MIS will need to acquire accurately all this information together with other details such as 'patient category' (e.g. private, NHS, Category II, etc.), in order to support a system of clinical budgeting adequately. Many laboratories, of course, make use of computers, often linking them directly to automated analytical equipment. In the larger systems computers process all laboratory requests, producing directly the clinicians' final reports. However, not all systems have ready-made Korner facilities as part of existing software. This means that, in order to use existing computer systems for Korner, either new and specific programmes for this purpose will need to be integrated with Present ones—which is not generally an easy task—or entirely new software will be required. Since there are five main branches of pathology, some with separately organised sub-branches, Korner implementation in pathology is likely to be a major undertaking with considerable capital and revenue implications.

Not all activity in pathology departments is as easily measurable as tests and requests. Consultations, teaching and various types of re-search activity are all recognised legitimate functions. As with work of the clinical psychologist or, say, domiciliary visits by community nurses, these activities are much more difficult to record. All involve a subjective element, necessarily employ self-recording and are open to bias favouring the recorder. Even the development of small personal computer-based recorders is unlikely to overcome these problems.

We believe that the particular difficulties in pathology are echoed in varying degrees in other health care service departments, many of which have yet to employ computer facilities. Where computers are adequately programmed it will be possible for the data to be correctly recorded since a 'request' or other required datum may be defined by the programme and not by the operator. Where this is not the case, districts will find it necessary to appoint data administrators, respon-sible for the purity of the data by policing the data acquisition protocol and facilitating the resolution of problems encountered with manual data collections. Overall responsibility for Korner implementation, however, remains with general managers and the rate of successful introduction will depend upon their skill and energy, helped no doubt by their desire to use better management information.

Databases

The term 'database' has acquired a special meaning. It is no longer appropriately applied to ordinary files of data, however comprehensive and voluminous these might be, even if they are held on computer storage 'media such as magnetic disc or tape. The term refers to a particular type of file structure which allows comprehensive data access to all the data, when required, for a variety of different purposes and, commonly, by different members of the organisation. It follows that data which might have been originally collected for a specific purpose would be stored in a database in such a way which separated it from that purpose, that is, independently, so that it then became accessible for any other legitimate organisational reason whether or not that reason was related to the original purpose.

For example, the age of each patient is routinely recorded as an essential part of the clinical function of diagnosis and treatment. Using a database, we might use 'age' to give information about the ages of patients in particular disease categories and their hospital referrals or some other index of health care consumption. We might choose to do this within social category or geographical location. We could express this information numerically and statistically test for significance any observed difference between age and social groupings. We might wish to use such information in building a predictive health needs model for our catchment area. The versatility of the database is illustrated by the fact that a simple file, be it manual or computerized, is only capable at any time of giving, as information, all or part of a single currently addressed record. On the other hand a database permits questions to be asked concerning certain common fields within all records held on file and either to give answers in numerical form or to identify file entries having specified characteristics.

A field may be regarded as a data item or entity within a record—the field on which a computer search may be made is referred to as a key. Examples of keys would include unit number, surname, etc. A data-base may be regarded as having many such keys. Indeed in many instances every field may be regarded in that way and a combination of keys may be specified to search for specific information. These are known as search parameters and vary with the sophistication of the database. The sophistication and power of the database is also related partly to the Database Management System (DBMS) which is the software that supports the database.

Advantages of the Database Approach

At first it was thought that the database approach would permit the establishment of very large databanks which would be capable of holding all the data relevant to an organisation. Centralization in this way would avoid duplication of data and of data entry with conse-quent cost savings. Moreover, data control and validation procedures would be improved, thus reducing inputting errors, whilst other important matters such as privacy, security, access to data and data redundancy would be subject to an organisational policy administered by a database administrator and his/her staff. Although there are obvious economies of scale in this approach there may be also wastage. As we have seen, information is a powerful resource which is fre-quently required instantly if its potential is to be maximized. Delays in either data entry or data access which may occur with very large systems reduce the effectiveness of the database approach and pre-dicate the need for systems tailored to local requirements. As with systems, there is a great deal of debate as to where to place the database boundary. This problem is compounded by the fact that databases may be operated on almost any computer, including micro-computers and personal computers, provided the required backing storage is of sufficient capacity. To narrow the breadth of the data items held is to negate the principal advantage of the database and it is a matter of judgement as to the point at which this trade-off with speed and access facilities best serves the interests of an organisation.

In health districts much patient data will be centrally held in a computer-based PAS and it will be possible for 'satellite' computer systems to access patient identification data from this directly. How-ever, in large multiple access systems there are particular security problems. Only certain data fields should be accessible to specified users so that confidentiality is maintained. This is usually achieved by specifying a hierarchy of access within the organisation. Some users will be permitted only to access certain fields of specific files while others will be cleared to update or 'correct' the information on file. Once new data is entered it is instantly and simultaneously available to all authorized users. Delays in information access are therefore likely to arise more from delays in data entry than computer function, even when the database operates as a real-time system. That is to say, the data is processed by the computer sufficiently quickly to appreciate and/or influence events as they occur. For example, patient identifi-cation data may be captured by the computer as part of the routine admissions procedure but not, say, during an emergency admission at night where it might be left until the morning for the computer clerk to enter. Details of transfers of patients between wards, consultants, or specialty care may be batched and left to be entered 'when there is time'. If the database is to be a working tool for the health care system it needs to be managed and operated efficiently, otherwise it will become discredited and poorly serviced by users of all kinds.

Computer Systems Design

At an early stage in their development computers were evaluated in terms of both their real and potential activities. Functions that could be computerized, it was thought, would relieve the tedium of manual data operation and 'speed things up'. In fact, initially, few processes were speeded up and tedium in work frequently arose as a consequence of computerization.

As computers became more sophisticated, emphasis in

systems design centred on the outputs the computer could provide which could effectively serve current organisational requirements. In specifying computer outputs to meet operational goals, specific data input re-quirements were identified. The systems designer, therefore, specified the process or programme functions within the computer necessary; to operate on inputs and produce the required outputs typically comprising reports, listings, computer files, etc. However, this process has been described as a 'dangerous practice' since the information require-ments of an organisation are never static. Although maintenance and evolution on a continuing basis are an integral part of the design process it has been found that prespecifying system outputs and building them into the system design can result in inflexible systems which are rendered obsolete by organisational change and which are therefore incapable of best meeting organisational needs. In theory this should not be a problem—but it is not a perfect world.

Data Analysis

Data analysis is an approach to systems design which seeks to alleviate the problems associated with organisational change. It is based not on any particular information requirement or function of an organisation but on the data from which such information may be obtained.

Data analysis within an organisation is undertaken as a quite separate and distinct activity from consideration of any hardware, computer or otherwise, that may be eventually employed to run the system. It assumes that data is a corporate resource, always to be shared between users and between applications and therefore must not be exclusively linked to any one of them. It implies that personnel within an organisation are not free to implement individual computer systems unless they both contribute to, and comply with, the data analysis specifications for the entire organisation.

In terms of stability, data will usually outlast the functions of any organisation. After some 40 years, several governments, three reorganisations and many changes, the NHS still has entities such as patients, doctors, tests, treatment sessions and so on, even though the recording of them and the use to which such data are put has changed over the years and is likely to continue to change. In the NHS, responsibility for data analysis resides with the NHS Corporate Data Administration (CDA) which works with users of all kinds to produce coherent and accurate data models for all NHS activity.

Data Modeling

Data models may be regarded as techniques for representing infor-mation and are, at the same time, sufficiently structured and simplistic to fit well into computer technology. In this sense a model is a basic system of constructs used in describing reality. Put simply, a data model is a jigsaw or map of all the pieces of information in the service and their relationship with each other but it is not a panacea. What it does provide is a broader corporate view of an organisation's information requirements before a lot of money is spent discovering that systems designers have not understood it per-fectly and have designed systems that are incompatible. Data modelling ensures that common terms used in different parts of an organisation are given standard definitions and, moreover, the implied relationships between the terms and the special characteristics associated with each term are identified. The key to data modelling is the identification of organisational entities. We may regard an entity as 'anything relevant to the enter-prise about which information could be or is kept'. Entities may be human such as 'patient', 'GP', 'consultant', or conceptual such as 'specialty', 'request', or geographical such as 'ward'. The CDA Korner Data Model contains 180 defined entities.

Use of the model ensures that wherever these concepts are used in any systems design the same definitions are applied. Similarly the special and important details about each defined entity, known as attributes, are also defined. Thus 332 attributes have also been defined to serve the Korner Data Model. For example, in the obstetrics model both the 'place of delivery'—and address, and 'presentation of the fetus before labour'—a clinical description, are attributes of the entity 'registrable birth'. In this way administrative and medical systems may be designed with inherent compatibility, the designers understanding all the attributes of all the relevant entities that may be needed by interacting systems.

The relationship between entities is denoted by a line. A simple line indicates a one-to-one relationship, whereas a triangular 'crow's foot' is used to indicate a multiple relationship. A full discussion of the theory and potential benefit of data model-ling is included in the *NHS Charter for Data Modelling and Data Administration* available from the CDA.

The Data Dictionary

Precise and agreed definitions are held in a data dictionary which may be regarded as being a reference source of data about data. For example, when considering the definition of the entity 'patient', are we to include persons who are unwell and self-administering their medi-cation though undiagnosed by a medical practitioner? A GP might accept this description, regarding all persons registered at his practice as patients, regardless of whether they have ever consulted him. If the definition is narrowed to that of a person suffering illness and under health care then the definition must be precise about when a person becomes a patient and when he ceases to be a patient in terms of the data model. The entity description for the entity 'patient' in the CDA Korner Data Model defines a patient as:

> '.. .a person with a specific disease or condition who receives treatment within the District. An entry on the patient master index. This may be a person who uses a hospital bed in order to receive clinical care/treatment or someone attending a clinic, day care facility etc. It will also include people in the community receiving care under a programme forming part of nursing care in the community. This also includes patients on the elective admission list who are awaiting elective admission.'

Common, agreed and precise data standards facilitate rapid, com-patible, systems design which may not only be independent in its function and choice of hardware but also in methodology. Given essential hardware compatibility, various computer systems and manual systems may interface harmoniously if they are based upon a common data analysis and data definitions.

Other Uses of Data Analysis

Data analysis should help in assessing which organisational operations require computer support and which tasks are better left as manual procedures. Computer applications packages may be evaluated using data analysis and boundary decisions regarding the size, location and funtion of databases, and the siting of, and access to, computers can also be assisted by this approach.

Applications Analysis

Systems analysis, that is the examination of organisational activity to determine how best the same objectives could be met with the help of a computer, can proceed independently of data analysis and will usually consist of functional analysis—finding out how the organisation operates and what is required—application design and programme development. Applications assumptions will include the design and creation of a database for all data required by the current applications and all others as they may arise. The concept of a corporate data model for the NHS is relatively new and many existing computer systems were implemented before it was described and made available by CDA. As a consequence of the data modelling approach it will no longer be acceptable for individual NHS computer users solely to define their own system requirements without reference to the model. Nor will it be sensible for commercial software suppliers, or NHS programmers, for that matter, to disregard the corporate data model. Local applications analysis and systems design will, in future, be required to be congruent and compatible with the model. Indeed, local analysts may well contribute ideas to the model. The CDA are committed to further development and may welcome such ideas and information regarding organisational change and development. Statements of systems requirements and detailed specifi-cations, therefore, should include compliance with the CDA data model, assuming a database configuration and specifying minimum requirements of the DBMS software.

Networking

By a computer network we usually have in mind a number of computers interconnected and intercommunicating in some way: that is to say without the need to transfer data or instructions manually between them. This definition may also be applied, though less charac-teristically, to computer terminals. If all the computers in a network are of a similar type and/or manufacture, then networking may be quite simple provided the computer hardware is able to comply fully with the network 'protocol'. Hardware 'incompatibility' between computers may be resolved by more sophisticated networks which, via connecting interfaces, convert data to a common form when entering the networks and to a specific form when leaving it. By this means it is possible to address computers of differing manufacture, size, configuration and complexity and to regard them as compatible.

Networks which are confined to a single building or a special group of functions are often designated as Local Area Networks or LANs. In these, computer operations may be shared in such a way as to ensure that no single computer becomes overloaded with work and therefore unacceptably slow in its operation. Individual computer malfunction does not threaten the viability of the whole network and computers may be exchanged and/or reprogrammed during normal network operations. Moreover, certain computers may be assigned specific functions in the network such as file handling, database management or on-line data acquisiton while one computer may act as a network 'host' or 'gatekeeper' to regulate communications between the various 'nodes' of the network. It is possible to envisage local area networks serving the require-ments of sub-systems within a health district. The district system might consist either of a large computer with many terminals and interfaces to other computers and LANs which would serve, for example, the community or outlying hospitals, or a central LAN with 'distributed processing' of district data and database management.

The Development Of Computer Technology

It is all too easily forgotten that computers are a relatively recent invention emerging in certain university departments after World War II as tools for mathematical research. The subsequent development of this technology, which has included the microchip, has put more computing power into today's pocket calculator than was available in those large valve-driven prototypes of the 1940s, such has been the phenomenal growth of this technology. There is much to suggest that we are still at an early stage in computer development and inevitably much of the experience gained so far in using computers in health care must be evaluated in the context of what is still a very young technology. There are two further areas in which we expect shortly to see enhancements. The first is in the sophistication of the computer. At the heart of the computer is the Central Processing Unit or CPU which logically obeys programme instructions to operate on inputs and/or stored data to produce outputs or other stored data. This must exist in all conventional digital computers be they large (usually referred to as mainframe), mini (smaller) or micro (smallest). Although the CPU is able to carry out instructions at nearly the speed of light it can only do so sequentially and it is capable of being overloaded by an overwhelm-ing number of tasks. This can occur if many terminals and other peripheral equipment are used simultaneously.

A network configuration effectively allows several CPUs to be brought into play and the computing tasks may thus be 'distributed' within an organisation. A further technique, known as multi-processing, consists of the grouping of several CPUs in a single computer, perhaps, say, one CPU per peripheral device with a further CPU in overall control. Both these approaches reduce overload and facilitate processing. These ideas have been considerably extended by the development of the Transputer which may be regarded as a multiple number of CPUs capable of working in parallel, i.e. simultaneously, on different por-tions of the same computer task. Since transputers are being developed using microchip technology we can expect to have ,very much more powerful desk-top transputer-driven computers in our networks in years to come. This, we believe, will greatly improve data accessibility and will in turn require a more dynamic approach to database management in health care.

The second area of development will concern the physical problems of data capture. Before entry into the computer memory all data *must* be converted into binary code. Where this at present involves the use of an on-line keyboard which is a very slow method of data entry, it has the potential to become a rate-limiting factor in computer operations. It also requires the operator to possess good keyboard skill.

This problem may be alleviated by a number of techniques. Optical Character Recognition can be used to input type scripted data and the use of pre-encoding, for example bar coding, may be helpful, particu-larly for standard handwritten information. For example, bar codes representing requests for investigations by service departments may be held in catalogue form in those departments to be read by laser or light pen on receipt of a corresponding handwritten request. Alternatively devices exist that permit direct entry of handwritten information Finally, voice technology may permit data entry to be effected in a 'hands off mode and by telephone.

Since many departments and sub-systems in the district require access to the same basic data, the elegant way to effect such access is by single, validated (error-checked) entry and accessible on-line storage within a database. It is possible to envisage issuing to patients a health card, similar in size and construction to a credit card which would magnetically (or optically) contain not only demographic information concerning the patient but a salient (perhaps recent) medical history or attendances record. The patient could register his arrival at the hospital or clinic by inserting his health card in a computer reader, the computer might then advise him of admission details or clinic waiting time, etc. The health card could be updated as part of the sequence of health treatment and be used as an identification device throughout the district, region or even the UK, being particularly useful in instances of accident and emergency. Such a philosophy presupposes the future implementation of extensive computer networking and/or wide distri-bution of compatible computers and terminals throughout health districts.

Long-Term Data Storage

Traditionally this has been achieved by the use either of printouts or by the storage of magnetic tape or disc. While magnetic tape is an economical storage medium by comparison with conventional filing systems it is a sequential medium requiring a computer to read it. This may be both an advantage and a disadvantage depending on the nature of an enquiry. Computer printout may be microfilmed or a microfilm output device may be interfaced as a computer peripheral for this purpose. Computer Output Microfilm (COM) is a particularly space-efficient storage medium and may be accessed manually, with speed, provided a satisfactory microfiche index is maintained. Such a medium has been used for the long-term storage of medical records in some districts and some departmental records also. However, such records are difficult to re-enter directly to the computer.

It is possible that records may in future be preserved on optical storage devices such as compact discs which are capable of holding much greater amounts of data per unit than either magnetic tape or microfilm. However, at present, like microfilm, compact discs cannot be conveniently updated and are only suitable for the archiving of medical records. The decision whether to use such media is one of systems design and is about the stage at which these records are to archived, e.g. on the death of a patient; or a move from the district; or merely a discharge from current treatment? Records so stored are regarded as permanent. Medical records held in this way would require transferring to the computer for updating during a treatment period and subsequently re-archiving in optical form on final discharge.

Privacy, Confidentiality and Protection of Health Information

Although they are separate issues, these three aspects of data control inter-relate and problems concerning them are exacerbated by the developing use of computers. For a discussion on the inter-relationship of these issues the reader is referred to the Lindop Report which predated the Data Protection Act by some 7 years, and to the more recent Korner report on confidentiality. Privacy carries with it the notion of being apart from company or observation—a place of seclusion and secrecy. In this sense privacy applies more to individ-uals or groups than to the data about them, the status of which is clearly contextually dependent. Different data items, though private to an individual, are often shared with different sections of society. For example, financial information with the bank manager, health infor-mation with the health worker, and usually neither of these with working colleagues or casual acquaintances. Lindop proposed the term data privacy to mean the individual's claim to control the circulation of data about himself.Privacy is an issue quite separate from the use of computers.Without reference to the computer, several unsuccessful private members' bills, presented to Parliament in the 1960s, sought 'to protect a person from any unjustifiable publication relating to his private affairs-and to give him rights at law in the event of such publications'. It was not until 1969 that bills were (again unsuccessfully) introduced which were concerned with computerized personal information.

The issue of confidentiality arises when there is a need

or wish to share data. In this sense 'ownership' of the data may be regarded as having been temporarily transferred to another person as may occur in exchange for some particular service, e.g. health service, on the understanding that it will in all other respects remain private infor-mation. (It should be noted, however, that strictly there exists no legal title to information as such, only to the storage medium, if any, that contains it. The term ownership is therefore used here subjectively.):

There appear to be three categories of personal health data. First, there is that which is necessarily shared with clinicians and others as part of the process of consultation; for example, the description of, symptoms, relevant personal details, life style, personal habits and even family history. Secondly, there is data which arises from medical activity. This is also factual data— the diagnosis, prognosis, the results of various tests and, particularly in psychiatry, the categorization of behaviour, addictions, phobias, etc. Although this constitutes infor-mation about an individual patient, the prerogative of 'ownership' has always been exclusively claimed by the medical profession on the basis that the regulation of health information is integral to the treatment process and that 'your secrets are safe with us'.

The third type of data is that which is gathered in the course of health work without the knowledge or even perhaps, against the will of, patient or client. It may be of a subjective or contentious nature, the clinician's or health worker's opinion expressed in contradiction to that of the patient, say, rather than straightforward medical obser-vation; the social worker's assessment of a client's living conditions and ability to cope, the likelihood of a child sustaining non-accidentatal injury from a parent or guardian and so on. It was argued by some respondents to the Lindop Committee that the more sensitive the data area, the less likelihood of it being computerized. While this may well be a valid assumption, generally, Lindop discovered systems which enabled a good deal of subjective data to be encoded and held in database format. In general, for all health data, as the Korner report on confiden-tiality has expressed, maintenance of confidentiality rests on ethical codes of practice for the professions, staff awareness and health authority procedures. The role of the Data Protection Act, 1984 in safeguarding confiden-tiality is expressed in the eight principles, particularly regarding the use and disclosure of personal data. However, the issue of data protection relates to wider considerations of accuracy, freedom from data corruption, unauthorized access and security.

The thrust of the Lindop report is that data accuracy should be verified by the data subject himself. In health care this would lead to greater accuracy, would moderate tendencies for capricious entries and help to remove suspicion that patients or clients may feel towards the use of computers. However, at the time of writing, the status of medical information and medical records in relation to the Data Protection Act is under national review. Database entry may in future occur from many sources in both community and hospital. Data protection strategies must guard against inaccurate data being entered and subsequently used for decision-making without verification. Precisely what is recorded and the entry and verification protocol will require to be controlled by locally agreed codes of practice and not solely by individual whim. Database access and the analysis of data for purposes other than those for which it was collected, a principal advantage of a database, is specifically prohibited by the Data Protection Act unless individual indentification data is removed from the records. Therefore, those with a need for database access may well be cleared to access specific data categories only, depending on status.

Data files would be segmented to exclude patient identification or other data fields from particular users and/or terminals.

The siting of data terminals themselves, to prevent operators being overlooked when accessing sensitive information, or unauthorized use of their terminals, could well be achieved by normal security measures and the locking of the office door. If, as is likely, large health computer systems are linked with the public telephone system, we may yet see attempts by computer 'hackers' to gain unauthorized access via other computers.

The consequences of such access to medical records could be far-reaching, particularly if their contents were changed or if their data were used for attempted blackmail of the patient. Subsequently, health authorities might face prosecution under the Data Protection Act for jack of security. There is also the problem of third party access to information as might occur through hardware or software mainten-ance and development by outside contractors. Finally, there remains the matter of data updating and the erasing of redundant data. Depending upon the size and scope of the database these functions may be prompted automatically. Heavy and prolonged caseloads will make it impossible for health workers to remember what information has been entered for each case. Under the current act Personal data held for any purpose or purposes shall not be kept for longer than is necessary for that purpose or those purposes.' A likelystrategy for complying with this requirement would be for certain data categories to be automatically deleted after the occurrence of certain events such as the final discharge of a patient or after a given period of time. Alternatively, the problem might be tackled by the application of an exclusion clause under the provisions of the Act.

It could be argued that any improvement in practice brought about by increased awareness; public pressure, and the Data Protection Act, should be supported by legislation extending to all data rather than only that held on computers and automatic processing equipment This matter was debated by Lindop and the matter was also subjected to a minority report. However, while further national legislation is unlikely in the near future it is open to health authorities to adopt the spirit of Lindop and Korner by accepting the recommendations of these Committees: that their principles be adopted as helpful guidelines to their own methods of data handling, both manual and computer-ized, and that they (health authorities) will make their own efforts to comply with them.

Index